CW00486394

The Entrepreneurial Patient:

A Patient's Guide to Hip Impingement

by

Anna-Lena Thomas

Thomas, Anna-Lena. The Entrepreneurial Patient: A Patient's Guide to Hip Impingement. 1st edition.

ISBN: 978-0-9886372-0-7

Editor: Ulf Buchholz

Reviewers: Dr. Chad Hanson and Jerry Hesch, PT, M.S.

Illustrator: Raushan Carter

Publisher: The Entrepreneurial Patient/Anna-Lena Thomas

This book is dedicated to my husband, David. Thank you for always being there for me — for better and for worse — and for encouraging me to write this book. You are my rock.

ACKNOWLEDGMENTS

A heartfelt thank you to Dr. Chad Hanson. This book came together much with help of your expertise as well as willingness to answer questions and review this book in its entirety.

My warmest thank you to Jerry Hesch, PT, M.S., for assisting with conceptualizing and reviewing the anatomy and rehabilitation chapters of this book. I am also grateful that you led me in the right direction to get treated for femoroacetabular impingement and labral tears.

I am thankful to have the unconditional love and support of my parents and especially my mom who doesn't hesitate to travel across the Atlantic to help my family.

Thank you to my friend and massage therapist Karina Braun for being a knowledgeable confidant in my medical quest and for encouraging me to write this book.

Thank you to my friend Sophie for always listening and offering both empathy and good ideas.

Thank you to my friend Cecilia who never hesitates to lend a helping hand or a listening ear.

Thank you to my friend Judy who inspired me to write this book and to its title.

CONTENTS

PROLOGUE

When, in November of 2010, I first came to the orthopedic surgeon who ended up performing both of my hip surgeries, I was talking frantically and presented him with all kinds of ideas from my own research of the previous seven years. This doctor could have ignored my situation. I was so used to doctors dismissing me with "I don't know what's wrong with you", proceeding to shuffle me off to the next specialist that I was convinced I only had ten minutes to get my message across. I knew something was wrong with my hip/groin, and I thought that something might be hip impingement. I was determined to find out: Was this doctor going to help me or not?

By the time I came to "my" surgeon, I had been to the Mayo Clinic three times, tried medical specialties ranging from dermatology (yes, even!), through endocrinology to rheumatology. Not to speak of all the orthopedic surgeons I had seen; I had gone through seven different physical therapists and completed hundreds of hours of physical therapy, all of which ultimately made me hurt more.

I had received virtually every type of spine injection you can imagine by from various pain specialists, been offered back surgery, narcotics, anti-depressants and nerve medications, all of which I declined. At great expense, I even tried prolotherapy (proliferative injections) of my sacroiliac joint ligaments. But nothing ever helped my pain.

During the time from onset of my pain in 2004, I had gotten married and had a baby. I had quit a full-time job in communications to work as an independent contractor so that I could influence my own workload; sitting in an office chair all day was too painful. As my almost constant pain was getting progressively worse, especially after pregnancy, I had to decrease my physical activity to a bare minimum. That alone was depressing. My self-image was one of an athletic girl who played ten years of soccer, swam competitively for most of my youth and later on hiked, ran and did aerobics. The sedentary lifestyle was not only taking a toll on my body but on my psyche as well.

When faced with the hurdles of the health care system understandably some patients give up and accept medication as their only option. Once enough medical professionals have told you that nothing is wrong with you, it becomes easy to internalize that message. As if it sometimes isn't hard enough to get an accurate diagnosis, making your way through the administrative labyrinth of our health care system can be a daunting task. You truly have to be a persistent and, indeed, an entrepreneurial patient.

I decided to write this book while rehabbing from the surgery on my left hip. My goal is to offer you not only my encouragement and experience, but a comprehensive resource on FAI. I have researched and conducted interviews to provide you with the facts and ideas you need to be an entrepreneurial patient throughout the diagnostic process, surgery, rehabilitation and beyond. In no way does this book attempt to provide specific and individual medical or insurance advice. Neither does it describe every detail of anatomy or surgery. I have learned a lot along the way. It is my hope that sharing my experiences, mistakes and successes over the past eight years can help you get on the fast track to feeling better.

Sincerely,
Anna-Lena Thomas, July, 2012

1 INTRODUCTION

"What is an Entrepreneurial Patient?" you might ask. The question is valid since an entrepreneur is normally someone who runs a business. Being entrepreneurial also means being creative and innovative — just the kind of characteristics patients need in today's world. An ocean of information is at your fingertips through the Internet. An entrepreneurial patient is someone who takes charge of his/her health care situation through his/her knowledge of medical conditions and insurance. The entrepreneurial patient does not accept a shoulder shrug for an answer, but keeps searching for answers to solve medical issues. The goal of entrepreneurial patients is to improve the communication with health care professionals and insurance companies to produce better outcomes for themselves.

This first book in the series of The Entrepreneurial Patient is primarily a book for patients who want a comprehensive source of information about hip impingement (femoroacetabular impingement or FAI), its treatments and implications. It also includes tips on health insurance issues that pertain to FAI. If you want to learn to master the health insurance system or health care system in general, look for new books in the series The Entrepreneurial Patient.

One of the main goals of this book is to make most aspects of FAI comprehensible to the general public and those affected by the condition. This entails translating the Greek and Latin that some doctors use into layman's terms and creating a comprehensive source of go-to information. The Entrepreneurial Patient: A Patient's Guide to Hip Impingement will take you through an overview of hip impingement, a simple hip anatomy lesson, tips for finding an FAI specialist, a discussion of the diagnostic steps, surgical and conservative treatment, as well as recovery, ideas for surgery preparations, multiple facets of rehabilitation, life after rehabilitation and injuries secondary to FAI.

This book includes a chapter on FAI and its implications on pregnancy for women with FAI who are struggling with the decision whether to get pregnant or treat their hip impingement first. Last but not least, you will find tips on how to deal with your insurance company in regards to FAI diagnostics and treatments. Information on recent FAI research and a doctor interview make this book an important resource if you are struggling to get an accurate diagnosis, and before you make a decision to have surgery.

Over the years, I have found that the more doctors I see, the more alternative therapies I try, the more people I talk to, the more research I do and the more medical lingo I learn, the better I'm able to communicate with people working in the health care sector — physicians, medical assistants, nurses, insurance representative, billing staff, authorization staff etc. — and the smoother the ride goes.

Thinking about how much time I have spent trying to cure my pain, is emotionally painful. I certainly wish I had spent less time. Nevertheless, I like to think of it as time I invested. Although the returns aren't monetarily measurable, having the least pain and best health you can is worth more than you can imagine while you are healthy. Pain doesn't become a nagging issue until it's chronic. Lack of energy doesn't pose a problem until you feel it. You cannot actually miss something you have and have always had. Maybe that is why it is hard for many people to be genuinely empathetic of other people's pain.

While we can feel bad or sorry for someone who has cancer, we cannot know all he/she goes through and how he/she feels. Although hip impingement is not a life-threatening condition, a similar challenge faces young people with (sometimes undiagnosed) hip problems. Young people with hip impingement look healthy, sometimes even athletic. It's hard to believe that they can be in constant and sometimes excruciating pain. Countless times I have been told "You are too young to have all this pain," by doctors and friends alike. Whenever I felt frustrated by it, I tried to remind myself that everyone has their own challenges, whether they are of a medical nature or not.

Despite my best efforts to stay positive, and not let my health situation dominate conversations and social gatherings, there have been a few low points when I needed to vent. I am very lucky to have wonderful family and friends who are empathetic and understand my modified activity level. Listen to what your inner voice tells you, and get rid of as many negative influences as possible. They drain you of energy — energy you need to handle work, children, fruitful relationships and, not the least, your health care.

I wish you much success in beating FAI. Know that it can be done! Let this book be your companion for the ride. You can be an entrepreneurial patient too.

2 MY STORY

I just had to write this chapter. This book would not be complete without telling you my story, but I also had to relieve my built-up frustration with the health care maze. Please learn from me and your journey can be better (shorter, cheaper, less painful) than mine. This is how it all started. In 2004, I suddenly started having pain on the right side of what I used to call my lower back. I had moved to the United States only one year and a half earlier, to finish my degree in communications and public relations at Pacific Lutheran University, and was searching for my first job in this country. I was fit, energetic, and excited about my future. It was completely puzzling to me that I suddenly, out of the blue, started having this weird pain.

I told myself that if only I got stronger and worked out more, the "lower back" pain would get better. Since time wasn't an issue for me, between résumé writing and interviewing I spent many hours at the gym. The crux was that I didn't get anwy better. Quite the opposite, my symptoms got worse, but not yet bad enough that I couldn't ignore them. Soon enough I started a new job. In quite some pain now, I counted the days until my health insurance would kick in. The day came, and I went to a chiropractor, thinking chiropractic adjustments might help as my back was probably just "out." Well, they didn't. Despite the pain, however, I was still able to be active and naively thought that exercise would cure my pain. So I ran, I hiked, and I did gym workouts like step aerobics, yoga and body pump.

At my new job, I met David who is now my husband. After a year of dating we were married in Sweden. When we returned to the U.S., my dad's words were quietly ringing in my ears that maybe I shouldn't work out so much if I had that much pain. Maybe my body was trying to tell me something. Within a month of coming back to the U.S., I was already working full-time. When I'd come home from work, I'd go for a run.

Then, in June 2005, at the gym with my husband for one of our many workouts, I challenged the elliptical machine. When I got off the machine, I immediately had a deep, excruciating ache in my right groin. I now realize that groin is a rather unspecific term. Despite all my youth spent in sports, I knew very little about sports injuries. We went home and I spent the weekend icing the almost unbearable pain. I had to roll and scoot myself out of bed. Did this make me go to the doctor? Oh no, after all, "people get injured from working out all the time."

I laid low for a while, and hoped the pain would go away. Six weeks later, I tried an elliptical again. It took no more than two minutes before my groin put me in agonizing pain again. That was the end of my active lifestyle and the beginning of my "career" in health care. Over time, my groin pain became less acute, but developed new patterns and settled in to become a chronic, nagging and ever-present pain that to this day flares up with modest activity, like swimming or chasing a toddler.

In the fall of 2005, I finally caved in and saw a doctor, a rehabilitation physician (PMR). He told me I was too young to have back pain, mostly ignored the groin pain, and sent me to physical therapy. Because my polycystic kidneys were coincidentally found on an abdominal CT scan ordered by a general practitioner, the physical therapist I saw didn't dare treating me properly until I had seen a kidney specialist. Getting diagnosed with polycystic kidney disease (PKD) was rather traumatic because PKD is a genetic, life impacting disease without a cure. I was devastated and set out to find out as much as I could about PKD. It took another two months to get an appointment with a kidney specialist, who told me "come see me when you need dialysis." Writing this book, in 2012, I am thankfully still not close to needing dialysis, but I surely have a different, more caring kidney doctor. By November of 2005, I had quit my job, and I have never held a full-time job since. Approaching Christmas of 2005, I went to see an orthopedic sports doctor. He said it must be my sacroiliac (SI) joint that is causing problems, and sent me off to more physical therapy. When that didn't help, but made me worse instead, he ordered a hip MRI (magnetic resonance imaging) arthrogram.

So far so good, but my insurance company refused to pay for the arthrogram portion of the MRI, that is, the injection of dye into the hip joint. When I came back to the doctor with the films in hand, he told me the MRI without the arthrogram was useless to him. But he didn't fight the insurance company on this issue. Instead, the insurance company wanted me to have a diagnostic injection with a local anesthetic in the hip joint. If the injection removed the pain in the groin temporarily, then the insurance company would cover an MR arthrogram of the hip joint. It's just that I had lots of soft tissue pain in the groin area, so when I got the injection, I couldn't tell if it helped with the pain in the hip joint.

Had I been an entrepreneurial patient at that time, I would have insisted on getting the arthrogram approved as well as the MRI and checked on the authorization before going to the imaging center. I learned that lesson the hard way. Back at the orthopedic doctor's office, I told the doctor the injection did not numb my pain. He then let go of the hip as a source of pain! Because I did not get an arthrogram MRI done at that point, I also didn't know that I had a labral tear (tear of the labral cartilage in the hip). If it had shown up on an MRI, I am sure I would have looked more persistently in the direction of the hip joint as the underlying problem. Instead, I went on a 5-year journey through the health care system.

The orthopedic doctor now started looking at the lower abdomen as the source of my pain. He knew that the problem started after an injury while working out, but because some of the pain presented as lower quadrant abdominal pain, predominantly on the right side, he decided to look for a hernia. Although he could not feel a bulge indicative of a hernia, the orthopedic doctor recommended an exploratory laparoscopy.

In April of 2006, I underwent an uneventful diagnostic laparoscopic surgery of my abdomen and pelvis performed by a general surgeon. The not-so-great memory from this surgery is that I couldn't lie down for days because surgery gas pressed on my lungs and prevented me from breathing. Not breathing is bad; so I slept in an armchair and walked living-room circles with our dog in tow, trying to rid my body of surgery gas. All inconvenience to no avail: The surgeon did not find a hernia. In fact, he didn't find pathology of any kind. However, he did suggest I go to a gynecologist since gynecologists are used to abdominal wall issues (yeah, they are used to slicing the abdominal wall open and pulling out babies...).

At this point, the orthopedic doctor didn't know what to do with me, so he told me to "go see a pain specialist." He sent me to a doctor down the street, which turned out to be the first of several go-arounds with pain specialists. My case was like gold to this pain doctor: I was dying to find the source of my pain; no one could find anything wrong with me, physical therapy made things worse instead of better, and my lumbar spine MRI showed ever so slight L5-S1 disc pathology. And so the injections started.

In and out of the surgery center, I received lumbar spine injections at every disc level. Despite my hopes, none of the injections gave me any pain relief for even a second. That didn't stop the pain management physician from proposing to perform nerve ablation surgery at L-5/S-1 because the aforementioned pathology was "the only thing visible on my MRI." I have to pat myself on the back for listening to my instincts and not agreeing to have the nerve ablation surgery. My reasoning was: Why perform a diagnostic injection if you are not going to use the outcome of that injection to diagnose a problem? No pain relief, no surgery. I was now an entrepreneurial patient in the making.

Following this set of injections, I was briefly at my wits' end before deciding to seek help at the Mayo Clinic in Scottsdale, Arizona, in the summer of 2006. Because of my polycystic kidney disease, I was able to get an appointment fairly easily. The kidney doctor at the Mayo Clinic was my first point of contact, and he referred me to various specialties within the Mayo Clinic. While the Mayo Clinic is a well-oiled machine, and it's truly a pleasure to receive health care there, the results were not satisfying. The physical med rehab doctor (PMR) only came up with more physical therapy and/or sacroiliac injections as remedies for my troubles. Back in Las Vegas, I went in for sacroiliac injections, which did not help.

I had had high hopes in going to the Mayo Clinic, but was now reaching a low point. So many injections, hours of physical therapy, multiple doctors and even exploratory surgery without a diagnosis. That's when I went to my gynecologist for my annual exam and brought up my troubles with him. He suggested I go see a chiropractor. I didn't think I had anything to lose. In retrospect, I know that the lower back and sacroiliac adjustments were not benefitting me, but led to increased hypermobility. The chiropractors thought I had suffered an adductor strain or tear from the injury in June of 2005, hence all the groin pain, snapping and clicking.

The chiropractor's team worked to break up scar tissue using the Graston® technique and did a lot of soft tissue work in addition to adjustments. At least, I felt that this doctor was really trying his best to help me instead of shrugging his shoulders. Having recognized my muscle and fascial adhesions, he recommended that I try a type of ball rolling therapy. I am thankful for that recommendation: One because ball rolling provides pain relief and, two, because the therapist has become a friend and a confidant in my quest for medical answers.

After about a year of chiropractic, I actually had more pain in the buttocks than before I started the treatments. I concluded that what I thought had been helping me was probably making matters worse. Clueless about how to proceed in searching for an answer, my husband and I went on vacation to Sweden. During one of my worst moments of pain during our vacation, I asked my husband to massage my lower back. He touched the nodule that I knew had been present over the right sacroiliac joint for years, a lipoma. As he pushed down on it, it hurt terribly and referred pain to the groin. Since we didn't have any other explanation for my "sacroiliac" and groin pain, the lipoma seemed as good as any.

I had often asked doctors if a lipoma could cause pain. The answer was always: "No, not unless it's pushing on a nerve." Back in the United States, I went to my general practitioner and asked the same question again. Suddenly I received a different answer: Absolutely, the lipoma could cause pain and refer pain, too, if you push on it. At the time, it seemed like a good idea to have it removed, especially because my biological clock was ticking, and I really wanted to resolve some issues before getting pregnant.

Surgery was quickly scheduled with a general surgeon, who suggested taking out the lipoma in her office with a local anesthetic. Out of all the mistakes I made, at least I got this one right. I said "no," and insisted on general anesthesia at the hospital. I asked the surgeon if there was any risk of hitting nerves during the surgery. Her answer was: "This is so superficial, and I will be nowhere near your nerve." As if there were only one nerve! It turned out that the lipoma was huge. In fact, at my follow-up appointment, the surgeon couldn't stop talking about how surprised she was at the size of that lipoma and at how deep she had to dig to get it out. But the pain in my buttocks and groin persisted.

With the lipoma out and no new avenues to pursue, my husband and I decided to try for a baby. After all, it's never a good time. Three months later, a little heartbeat was visible on an ultrasound. On the sunny side, among all my medical issues, getting pregnant was never one of them. I had not given up getting better, but pregnancy put these efforts on hold. My pain in the buttocks escalated early in pregnancy, as did the burning pain around the hip and the groin pain as well as the clicking and locking and getting stuck of the hips.

Sacroiliac pain is nothing unusual in pregnant women. Combined with my undiagnosed hip impingement and the labral tears, the aches and pains were almost unbearable. By the time I was six months pregnant, I would have to stop in the middle of a step because of excruciating pain. That's when I once again started physical therapy. For once, the physical therapy actually helped put me back together. It didn't take away the pain, but at least the grinding of the sacroiliac joints stopped.

Approaching the end of pregnancy, which in other ways was perfectly normal and healthy, we found out that the baby was breech (butt down instead of head down). To this day, I don't know if that was a blessing or a curse. I didn't want to have anything to do with the c-section that I was ultimately forced into, but who knows how the labral tears would have been impacted by a vaginal delivery and how I would have held up considering my already significant groin pain.

Pain-wise the time following birth was rough, and the unavoidable lack of sleep didn't help. Coming off pregnancy escalated my symptoms, and added new problems unrelated to hip impingement, which further distracted my doctors from the main problem. Finding help got even more complicated. Almost immediately after giving birth, my left ankle fell apart, causing acute pain, and making it hard just to walk around the house. A few cortisone shots later, I could at least function.

Three months after the baby's arrival, I started looking for answers to my pain again. This time around, I turned to an orthopedic back doctor to get an MRI of my lumbar spine, since the lower back is where I felt a lot of pain after pregnancy — or at least that is how I defined the pain. After another round of physical therapy without improvement in symptoms, I "qualified," as my insurance company put it, for a lumbar spine MRI. Showing more protrusions than two years earlier, but nothing significant enough to warrant any invasive treatment, the doctor sent me out for even more physical therapy in the form of "an aggressive core stabilization program."

Going to this new physical therapist proved a turning point. No PTs before him had actually paid attention to anything I said, like "this lower abdominal exercise with hip flexion really hurts my hip and groin." To me, it seemed like that would have been useful information. My hip would clunk, catch and snap. For the first time ever, I heard the words: "I think you might have hip impingement." So I went home and researched everything I could find about FAI — a lot less information was available in 2009 than in 2012. Down to the least detail, the symptoms of FAI described in my research fit my pain. Now it was just a matter of finding a doctor to diagnose it. My physical therapist recommended a hip doctor at the same orthopedic center where the back doctor worked.

The orthopedic back doctor wanted to start a round of diagnostic injections of my lumbar spine. Here we go again! I told the doctor's physician's assistant (PA) that I had enough, and asked for a referral to the hip doctor who had been recommended to me. The PA told me "the doctors don't like losing their patients to other doctors within the group." That just blew my mind. Sorry Mr. Backdoctor, I'm out of here! Working my way toward entrepreneurial patient status, I drew the conclusion that revisiting fruitless routes were not worth my time or my money.

Luckily, my insurance didn't require a specialist referral. A couple of weeks later I went to the hip doctor's office hoping that my troubles were soon going to be history. I felt so sure of what my diagnosis would be that it completely caught me by surprise when, after his examination, the hip doctor said: "I don't think you have hip impingement. You have good range of motion." The x-rays didn't show any clear evidence of hip impingement either, "just a little overhang on the left socket." Well, I now know that's called pincer impingement.

Nevertheless, the hip doctor did order an MRI arthrogram of the hip. After all this time, and all the images that had been taken, this was the premiere for the hip MRI arthrogram. Bracing myself, I picked up the imaging report before I went to the doctor's office. It read labral tear. Imagine my surprise when the doctor told me that a labral tear was nothing we should or needed to treat with anything other than physical therapy. As for all the myofascial (soft tissue) pain that I had, the doctor suggested that I have a rheumatological condition. That's where he told me to look further.

Of course, I shouldn't have accepted that answer. Of course, I should have trusted my gut instinct that there was a problem in my hip. To my defense, this hip doctor was supposed to be about the best Las Vegas had to offer in terms of hips, knees and shoulders. Luckily our medical community has expanded since then. I should have researched doctors specialized in hip impingement, right then, and travelled to see one of them for a second opinion. An orthopedic doctor is not automatically qualified to diagnose FAI. I assumed this orthopedic doctor knew what he was talking about. I was wrong, and I have learned from it that not every orthopedic doctor is trained and qualified to diagnose and treat FAI.

The orthopedic hip doctor's suggestion to look at rheumatology sidetracked me and further delayed my hip impingement diagnosis. My husband and I decided that I should try travel to the Mayo Clinic again, this time to Rochester, Minnesota. I got this awesomely cheap read-eye flight — I thought — only to discover, just as I was about to board the plane, that my ticket didn't read Rochester, MN, but Rochester, NY. A snooty flight-attendant, $350 and four hours later, I was lucky to board the right connecting flight to Rochester in Minnesota. What was I thinking, traveling there the first week of January anyway? At least, I didn't show up at the hotel shuttle in flip-flops like some Floridians did — what were they thinking?

Sleep-deprived, I made it in time for my first appointment with the polycystic kidney disease specialist at the Mothership of Health Care. The Mayo Clinic is truly impressive. You get a schedule, and, like a school kid with a backpack, you trek through gigantic hallways and buildings full of all the medical specialties you can imagine. The efficiency is tremendous and the experience almost frustration-free. Was this where my mystery would be solved?

The kidney doctor at the Mayo clinic did a real thorough exam, and sent me out to various specialties and for testing. X-rays of my pelvis and lumbar spine came back showing sclerosis in the sacroiliac joints, and the blood work revealed a slightly elevated C-reactive protein level, an indication of increased inflammation in the body. These two findings were enough, in lieu of other ideas, for the kidney doctor to send me to the Mayo Clinic's rheumatology department. Unfortunately, there were no available appointments for a long time, so I flew back to Las Vegas and saw a local rheumatologist.

Back at home, the rheumatologist ordered a pelvis MRI (which provides a clearer picture than an x-ray), which came back completely "unremarkable" — no sign of sclerosis in the sacroiliac joints — and a whole battery of rheumatologic blood tests. Every single test, even the C-reactive protein, came back normal. Not a single gene for rheumatoid arthritis, lupus or ankylosis spondylitis (inflammatory disease of the joints between spinal bones and sacroiliac joints) was to be found. While that was a very good thing, where would that knowledge lead me? The rheumatologist hinted toward fibromyalgia and suggested I start taking Lyrica® (pregabalin, a medication used to treat neuropathic pain) and see a pain specialist. Here we go again!

Really — a pain specialist — is that what I had boomeranged back to? I decided to go and give one more pain specialist a try. The guy was a complete joke and told me that "our bodies aren't perfect". Maybe I don't need to tell you that I didn't go back. Springtime came around, and I decided to go back to the Mayo Clinic. This time I got an appointment at their spine clinic and rheumatology department. The spine surgeon looked at all of my medical records, and said he couldn't find anything wrong with my spine. He told me it seems like the pain is in the sacroiliac joints, around the hips and in front of the thighs. He then almost immediately started talking about fibromyalgia: "You know, that's a real condition." The next day, in the rheumatology department, the fibromyalgia expert thankfully concluded that I didn't meet criteria for fibromyalgia. Thank you so very much!

Next on the schedule was a sacroiliac joint injection, which I was quite skeptical of because it wasn't my first, but I agreed to go ahead with it "for completeness sake." Not surprisingly, the steroid injection didn't give me any pain relief because the problem wasn't inflammation. The injected anesthetic didn't do anything for me either.

From my research, I had found out about an anesthesiologist who started a Mayo Clinic clinical trial on prolotherapy of the sacroiliac joints. He was actually in clinic on my last day at the Mayo Clinic and willing to see me. He felt that pelvic instability might be my problem, because of all the unsuccessful physical therapy, the correlating myofascial symptoms and all the conditions that had been ruled out. To him prolotherapy was not experimental, although, insurance companies like to say so because they don't want to pay for it. The anesthesiologist told me that the results of the clinical trial were pointing toward good results when prolotherapy of the sacroiliac joints is combined with a physical therapy program for core stabilization. All the patients enrolled in the clinical trial had, just like me, done extensive core strengthening without the desired results of pain relief in the sacroiliac joints prior to starting prolotherapy.

At this point, I was convinced prolotherapy would be it. Back in Las Vegas, I did research to find a medical provider and yet again decided to go out of state. In California, I found a doctor of osteopathy (DO) who specialized in prolotherapy. Of course, my insurance company wouldn't cover these injections, so the treatments came at considerable expense to us.

After four visits to the California doctor for platelet rich plasma (PRP) injections into the ligaments of the sacroiliac joints, I came to the conclusion that the injections just weren't working, and there was no point in getting any more.

During the whole treatment course, I had diligently done my physical therapy with a therapist who was, anecdotally, "good at SI joints." I complained to her that neither the prolotherapy nor the physical therapy was working. The physical therapy — squats on a balance board, hip rotations and oblique curls with hip flexion among other exercises — would make me hurt more. Like so many before her, the physical therapist, who really poured her energy into getting me better, didn't know what to do with me other than suggesting more of the same.

I decided to switch it up. After some more research I found a physical therapist, surprisingly right here in Henderson, Nevada, who had a different approach to sacroiliac joints: The Hesch Method of Manual Therapy. In his research and practice of over 30 years, Jerry Hesch has developed a new understanding of the pelvis and the sacroiliac joints and as well as a treatment protocol that doesn't resemble the typical muscle energy techniques that physical therapists typically use to treat sacroiliac pain (1).

The Hesch Method is also non-traditional in that it does not require the patient to come for treatments two or three times per week for months on end. Contrary to the standard physical therapy schedule, the Hesch Method really is a short protocol for examining and treating joints and examining how joints co-function. A multi-step process where the result of one joint examination and/or treatment will generate the next step makes up this approach.

I decided to go through with the Hesch Method to see if it could cure my sacroiliac pain. At this point I would have done almost anything. It was either the Hesch Method or pixie dust. It didn't cure my sacroiliac joint pain, but it also didn't leave me with a shoulder shrug. Instead, I now felt confident that the sacroiliac joints themselves were not the root cause of my problems. In addition to evaluating my joints, the physical therapist looked over all my records and told me: "If it was just your sacroiliac joints that were the problem, I would have figured it out and treated it by now. But look here: labral tears in your hip joints - you have pathology in your hips. That's what I would go after, if I were you." Although I felt like I had already been there and done that, I decided to take a new stab at the hip issue.

At this point, it wasn't the first time that I had come across the words hip impingement. Things started happening quickly now. After some more research, I found out that there was a new doctor in town — a specialized arthroscopic hip surgeon named Dr. Chad Hanson. The orthopedic clinic's website read that Dr. Hanson had completed a fellowship program at The Steadman Clinic in Colorado with Dr. Philippon. That name was not new to me and I knew that Dr. Philippon is a huge name in the world of hip arthroscopy and hip impingement. Wasting no time, I made an appointment for the following week. Having learned a few things on my journey through the health care jungle, I checked the doctor's references by calling the Steadman Clinic in Colorado, where the Fellowship Director confirmed that their clinic stands fully behind Dr. Hanson's skills in hip, shoulder and knee arthroscopy.

With fresh wind in my sails, six years after the onset of pain, I felt hope that I was finally on the right track. Diagnosing my FAI was still not easy. It took four different diagnostic components, each one adding a little bit more information. There was no 100 percent certainty about the extent of my hip condition before I came out of surgery. The night before my first hip surgery, I slept poorly and dreamed that I woke up from anesthesia only to hear the surgeon tell me: "Sorry, you don't have hip impingement." Believe me, that was not a dream to me, but a nightmare. But, after I woke up from the 4-hour long surgery, and was still drowsy from the anesthesia, my surgeon came over to check on me. My first words were: "Did I have it?" As odd as it sounds, the answer, "Yes, you did", was like sweet melody to my ears.

In a bizarre way, after all those years of uncertainty and pain, I was actually happy to have (had) hip impingement. The surgery was only a beginning not an end. Now, my journey through the rehabilitation started. The FAI surgery has been beneficial to me as you will see in the chapter My Story – Continued later in the book.

3 AN OVERVIEW OF HIP IMPINGEMENT

The fancy name for hip impingement is Femoroacetabular Impingement (FAI). The hip joint is a ball-and-socket joint where the "ball" is the (femoral) head of the thighbone (femur). It rests inside the "hip socket", called the acetabulum. Together the ball and the socket make up the connection of the thighbone to the pelvic bone (for more information on hip anatomy see Chapter 4: Basic Hip Anatomy).

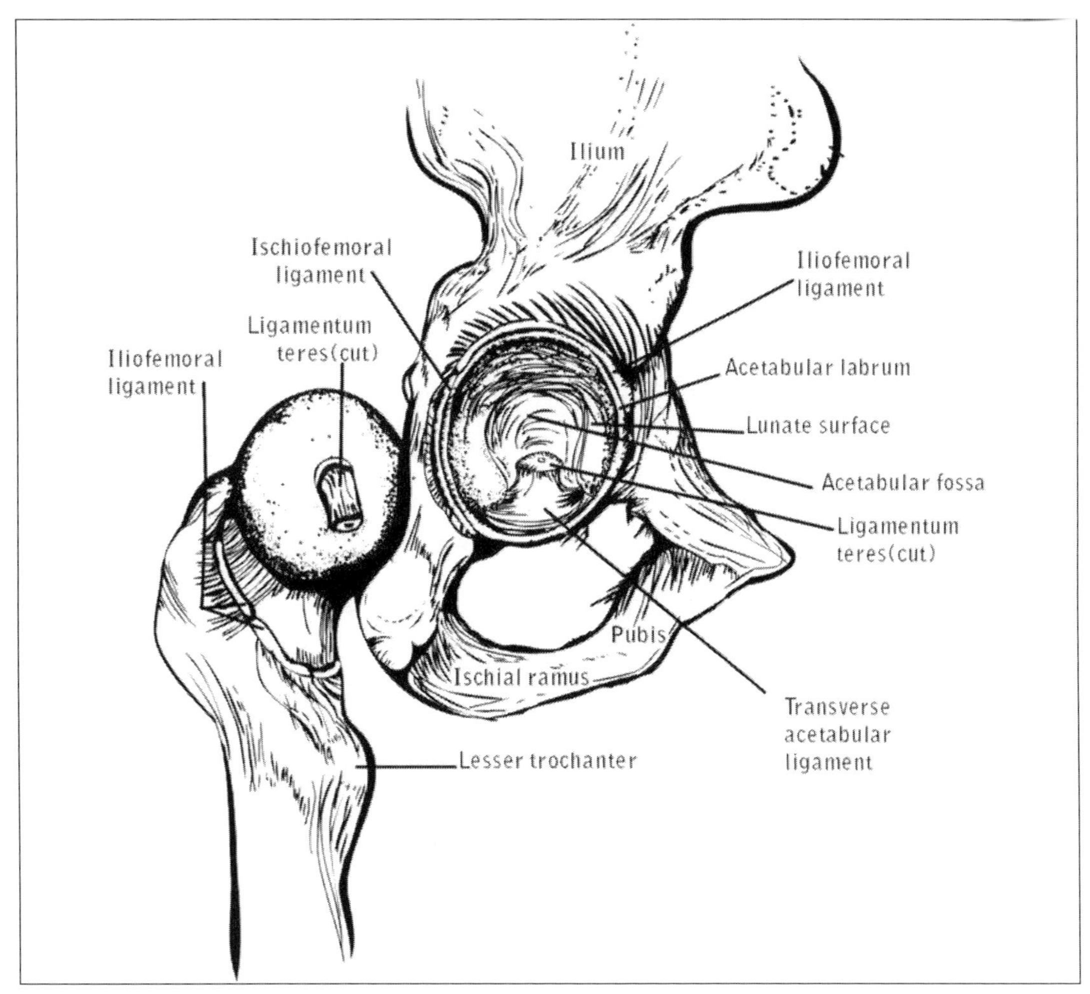

Figure 1: The right hip joint opened to show its internal anatomy

The illustration is modified from figure 12-13 in Donald A. Neumann's book *Kinesiology of the Musculoskeletal System*.

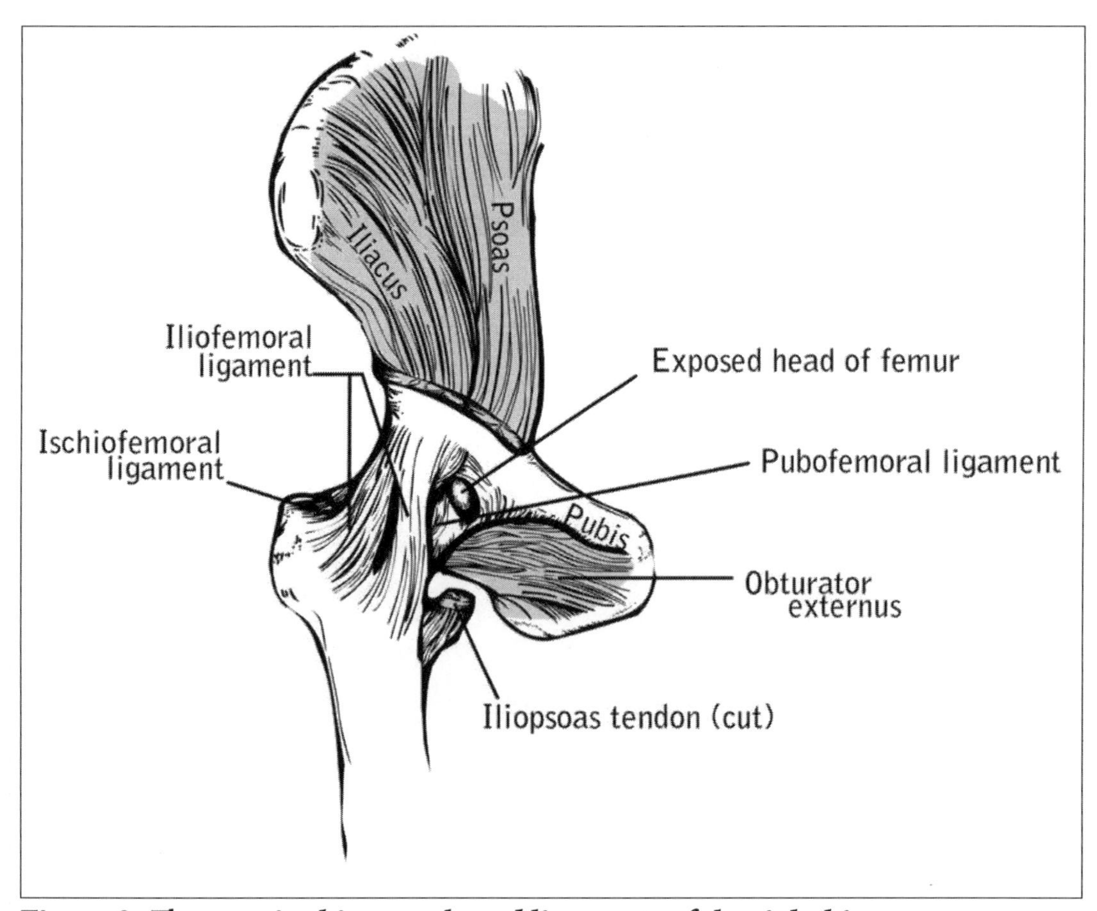

Figure 2: The anterior hip capsule and ligaments of the right hip
The illustration is modified from figure 12-17 in Donald A. Neumann's book *Kinesiology of the Musculoskeletal System.*

The CAM lesion consists of a bony "bump" on the ball (femoral head) or neck of the thighbone. Statistically, CAM lesions are the most common in young, athletic men. In a 2007 study that included 301 patients with diagnosed hip impingement on one side only, 100 (33 percent) of the patients, who were all treated arthroscopically, had isolated CAM impingement (3). *See Figures 4 & 5.*

In doctor's lingo, CAM can be described as "decreased femoral head neck offset" because there is extra bone on the neck of the thighbone so that the distance to the socket is decreased and the labrum gets pinched. The contact of the ball against the socket is most evident in flexion, adduction and internal rotation of the hip (for an explanation of the terminology see Chapter 4: Basic Hip Anatomy). That movement causes abrasion of the cartilage in the socket with pulling and/or tearing away from the labrum and the tip of the thighbone where there is also cartilage. This can lead to separation of the cartilage (4).

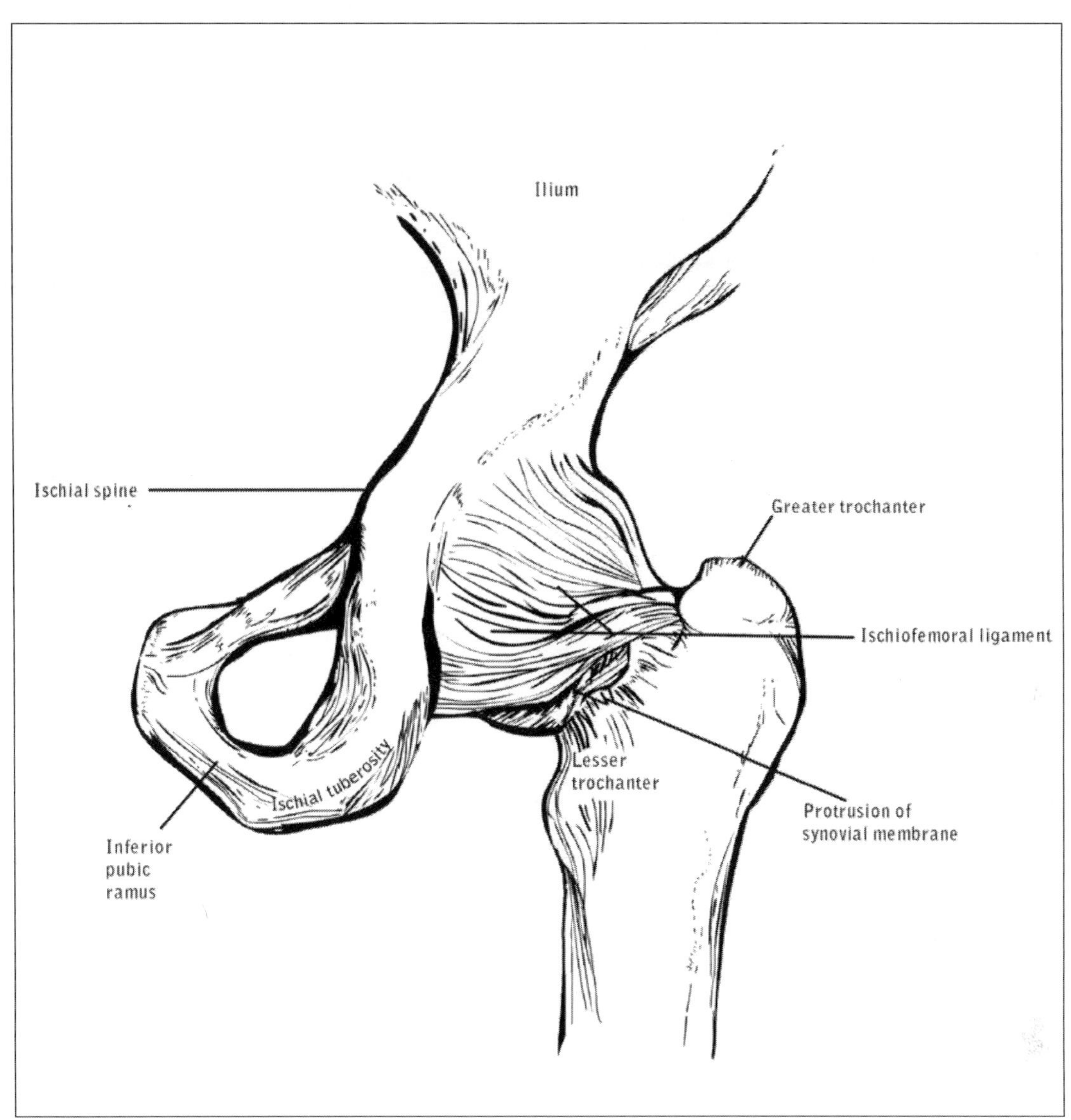

Figure 3: The posterior hip capsule and ligaments of the right hip
The illustration is modified from figure 12-18 in Donald A. Neumann's book *Kinesiology of the Musculoskeletal System.*

The most extreme — and quite rare — variation of CAM impingement is the "pistol grip" deformity. In this type of impingement, the junction between neck and head of the thighbone is convex instead of concave (5).

3.2 Pincer

A pincer lesion is caused by bone overhang or overgrowth in the hip socket (acetabulum). Pincer lesions are more common in middle-aged active women. Several abnormal shapes of the hip socket may lead to pincer impingement: coxa profunda, acetabular (socket) protrusion and acetabular retroversion (3).

Coxa profunda and acetabular (socket) protrusion are similar, meaning that the hip socket is too deep, but there are anatomical differences (see chapter 13 Glossary for definitions). Socket protrusion is the more uncommon variation of FAI. Despite anatomic differences, coxa profunda and acetabular protrusion are functionally the same and create the same problem — a problem that may lead to pincer impingement. *See Figure 6.*

Acetabular retroversion refers to the rotation or tilt of the front of the hip socket as it relates to the back of the hip socket. When doctors look at an x-ray for acetabular retroversion it is called checking for a cross-over sign, which compares the front and the back of the socket and measures the angle. It's imperative that the physician takes the tilt of the pelvis into account when looking for retroversion. If the pelvis is tilted the result of measuring the angle, the cross-over, might be skewed. If acetabular retroversion is present, it may also lead to pincer impingement (6). *See Figure 7.*

Spine conditions like scoliosis (abnormal curvature of the spine) or kyphosis (abnormal rounding of your upper back) can cause rotation of the pelvis, pelvis tilt and so-called functional retroversion of the hip socket. Similar to acetabular retroversion, functional retroversion also refers to the alignment of the front and back of the hip socket. However, it is not caused directly by an abnormal shape of the hip socket, but by other conditions. Prior thighbone fractures or surgery to cut and reshape the pelvis to correct hip dysplasia can also cause pincer impingement (4).

In the above mentioned study of 301 patients who underwent arthroscopy to treat FAI, 50 (16.6 percent) of the patients presented with, and were treated for, isolated pincer impingement (3).

3.3 Mixed CAM and Pincer

A pincer lesion is caused by bone overhang in the hip socket.

Not infrequently people with hip impingement do not have just one type of lesion but a combination of both — called mixed CAM and pincer. In these instances, there is both a bump on the neck/ball of the thighbone and overhang from the hip socket. In the literature, opinions seem to differ on how frequent CAM and pincer co-exist. Some physicians argue that CAM and pincer very rarely occur in isolation and that the most common type of FAI is a combination of CAM and pincer with CAM at the front of the neck of the thighbone and pincer at the front rim of the hip socket (4). The Philippon study cited above, found that 151 of the 301 study patients (just over 50 percent) had a mixed CAM and pincer impingement (3).

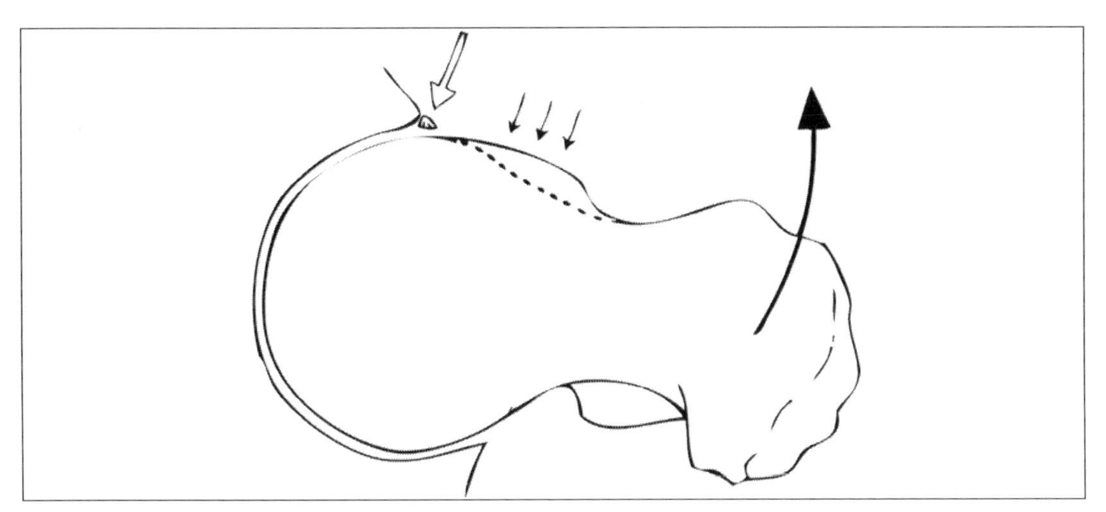

Figure 4: CAM lesion

The three black arrows point to the CAM lesion. Printed with permission from the *Journal of Bone and Joint Surgery American*, May, 2006, 88, 5, Treatment of femoro-acetabular impingement: preliminary results of labral refixation, Espinosa, 925-935.

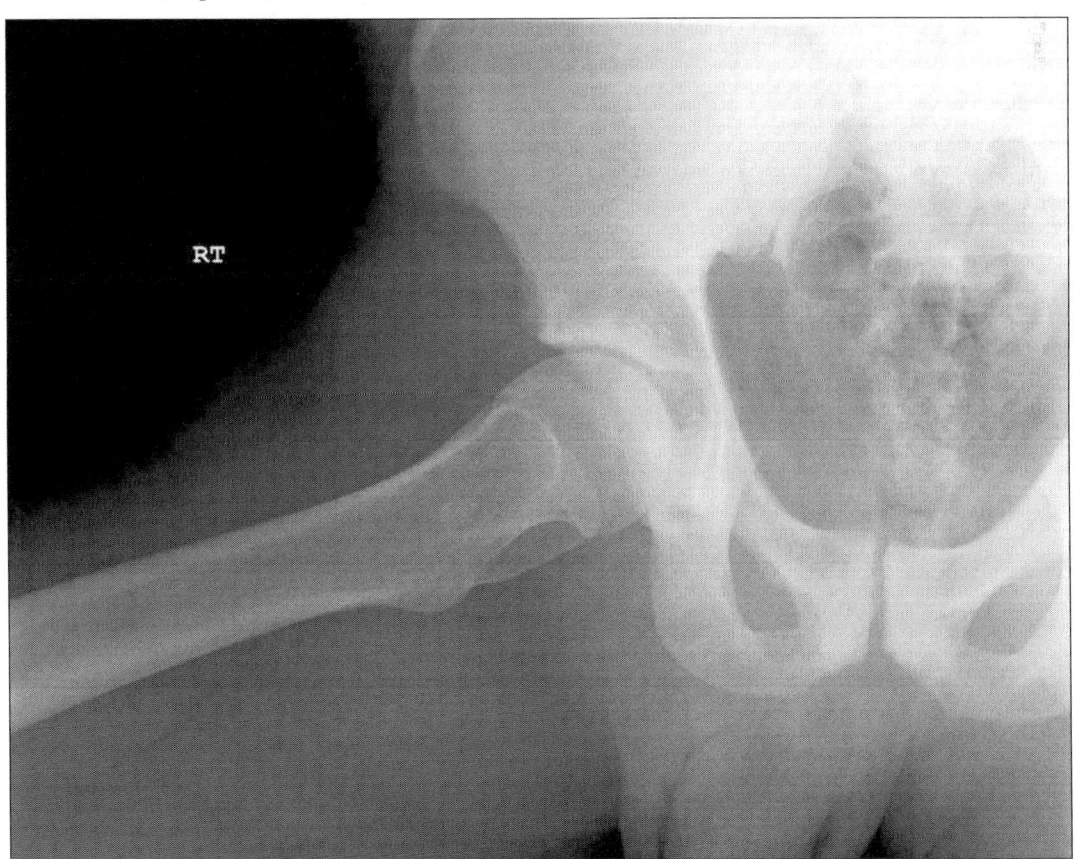

Figure 5: X-ray of CAM lesion in the right hip

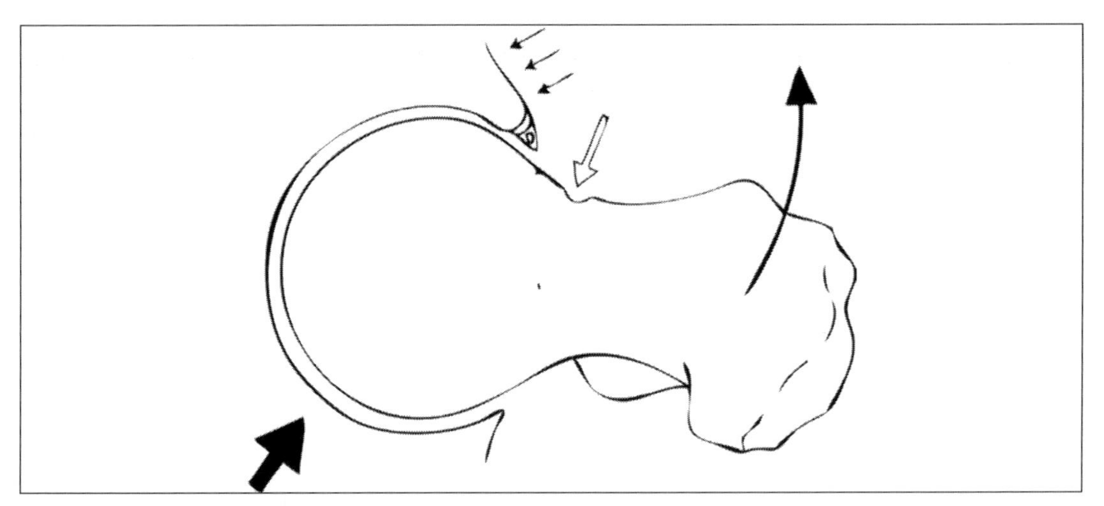

Figure 6: Pincer lesion

The three black arrows point to the pincer lesion. Printed with permission from the *Journal of Bone and Joint Surgery American*, May, 2006, 88, 5, Treatment of femoro-acetabular impingement: preliminary results of labral refixation, Espinosa, 925-935.

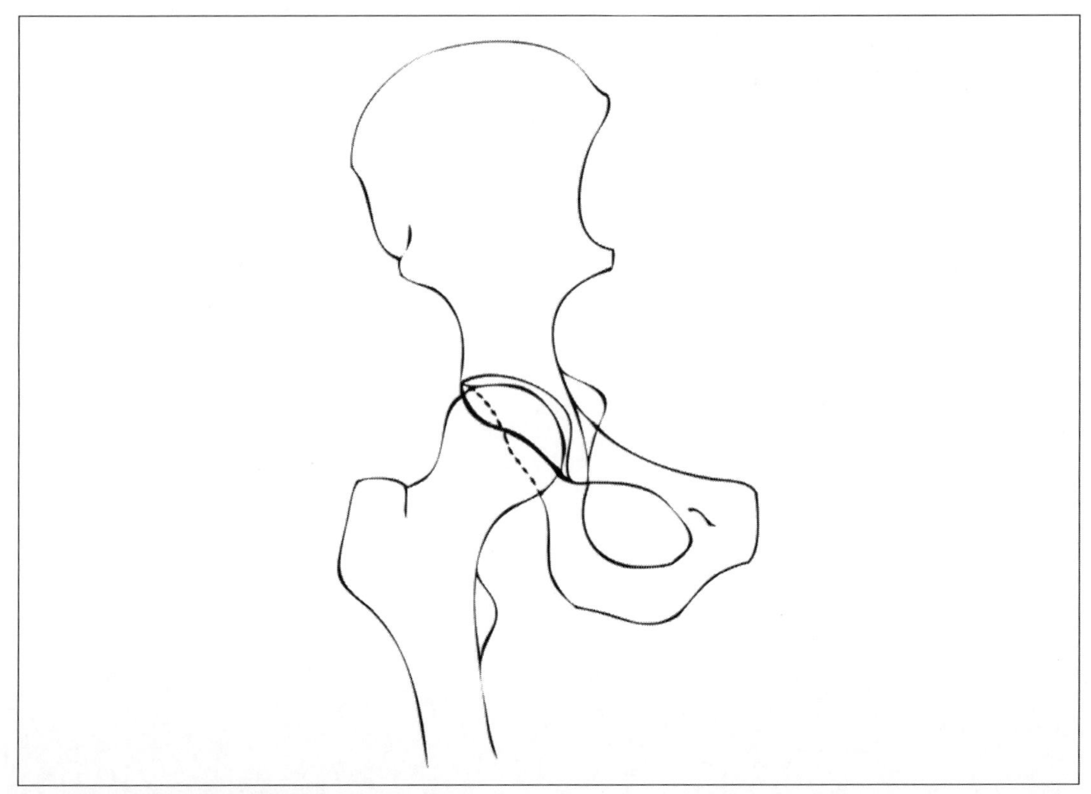

Figure 7: Acetabular retroversion

Printed with permission from the *Journal of Bone and Joint Surgery American*, May, 2006, 88, 5, Treatment of femoro-acetabular impingement: preliminary results of labral refixation, Espinosa, 925-935.

From a patient's standpoint, the surgeons' arguments don't matter. What matters is that you find a surgeon who can diagnose both CAM and pincer lesions, and is competent to remove them. In general, CAM lesions are better understood and easier to treat than pincer lesions. However, the pincer lesions should not be ignored during surgery, since they also lead to labral tears.

4 BASIC HIP ANATOMY

The hip joint is very complex with many attached muscles performing different functions, like hip flexion, extension, abduction, adduction and rotation. To confuse matters even more, some muscles may perform more than one task. A muscle that may be categorized as an adductor, for example pectineus, may not have adduction of the hip as its sole function but may also work as a hip flexor. Because hip impingement patients often struggle with muscle imbalances, it may be useful to understand some of the hip anatomy and its muscle dynamics.

A better understanding of the muscles can aid the physical therapy process and allow you to actively participate in finding and treating muscle imbalances. It can also help you communicate better with your doctor(s) regarding injuries secondary to FAI. I will briefly describe and define some foundational concepts of muscle movement and explore the major muscle groups involved with the function of the hip.

When you think of muscles, it's important not to think of them as singular entities, but as groups of muscles that work together to perform movements. Kinesiology is the science of human movement and large textbooks have been dedicated to this topic. Movement is not a simple concept to explain and understand. Central to our understanding of muscle movement is the frame of reference in which a movement occurs. In other words, it is important to describe what position the body is in when performing a certain movement: sitting, lying on your back (supine), lying on your stomach (prone), standing, bending, squatting, etc. Then, when you talk to a health care professional, you can mention a position to create a frame of reference for what is happening in the joints.

4.1 Movement Terminology

In anatomy, everything is based on a frame of reference and body position. In kinesiology it gets a lot more detailed than just referencing a position, like standing. Kinesiology's complex body reference system includes the three main planes and three axes when referring to specific body movements.

4.2 Planes and Axes

Planes are flat surfaces that are used to map three-dimensional space. To picture a plane, imagine a flat rectangle cutting through the body in a certain direction. Three major planes divide the body into sections: Upper and lower half (transverse plane), left and right side (sagittal plane), and front and back (coronal or frontal plane). Minor planes are slightly offset at an angle to the major planes. The major planes describe the body seen from an anatomically (neutral) position, meaning that the body is facing straight ahead with arms hanging down and palms facing forward. Each plane is divided by a major axis. An axis is an imaginary line around which a body part moves, similar to how the wheels of a car rotate around an axis.

The sagittal plane divides the body into left and right portions (imagine a line cutting through the middle of the head, navel and spine, between the legs and feet). The axis for sagittal plane movements of body parts is oriented side to side (horizontally) and described as the mediolateral (from midline-to-side) axis. Flexion and extension of the hip take place in the sagittal plane (7).

The frontal plane divides the body into anterior (front) and posterior (back) portions. The axis for the frontal plane is oriented front-to-back and is called anterioposterior. Abduction and adduction of the hip take place in the frontal plane (7).

The transverse plane divides the body into upper and lower portions. Those portions are in turn divided into superior (above) and inferior (below), or proximal (closer) and distal (farther away). The axis of transverse plane movements is oriented up and down and is

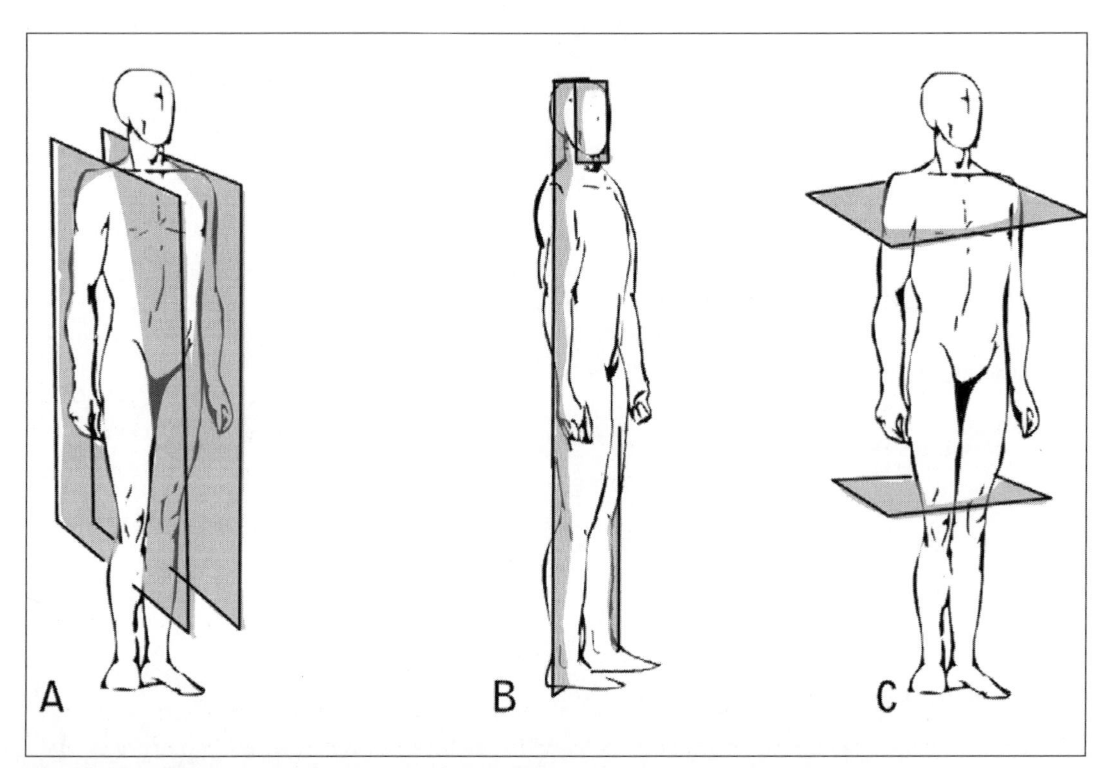

Figure 8: Planes and axes. A: the sagittal plane. B: the frontal plane. C: the transverse plane.

The illustration is modified from figure 1-4 in Donald A. Neumann's book *Kinesiology of the Musculoskeletal System.*

described as superior-inferior or simply vertical. Internal and external rotation takes place in the transverse plane (7). *See Figure 8.*

4.3 Basic Concepts of Location

The following concepts are used throughout medicine to describe location. Although the root meaning is the same throughout all medicine, the science of movement uses these terms to describe movement. I will provide descriptions that apply both to medicine in more general terms and to movement of body parts.

Anterior: Front or movement to the front.

Posterior: Back or movement to the back.

Medial: Midline, in the middle, or closer to an imaginary (sagittal) plane that divides the body into left and right halves.

Lateral: Side, on or seen from the side, or farther from the sagittal plane that divides the body into left and right halves.

Superior: Above or movement toward the head.

Inferior: Below or movement away from the head.

Proximal: Closer to something.

Distal: Farther away (distant) from something.

4.4 Basic Concepts of Movement

Before we explore the muscle groups of the hip, it makes sense to explain the concepts that give names to muscle groups and individual muscles. The following concepts are used to describe movement of muscles and are also used to classify muscle groups. They also apply to body parts other than the hip, like the shoulder, but for our purposes I will refer to the hip.

Adduction: "Add" means toward the midline of the body. Adduction of the hip means moving the thighbone (femur) toward the midline of the body.

Abduction: "Ab" means away from the midline of the body. Abduction of the hip means moving the thighbone (femur) away from the midline of the body.

Rotation: A circular movement of the hip joint. Rotation is divided into internal and external rotation. Sometimes internal rotation is also called medial rotation and external rotation called lateral rotation. It sounds simple, but, when you start looking at various body positions, distinguishing between internal and external rotation can sometimes be confusing. Just keep in mind that both internal and external rotation refers to the rotational direction of the hip joint in relation to the position of the thighbone.

Internal rotation is a twist of the hip joint (thighbone) inward, for example, pointing your toes in toward the middle of your body. You can perform internal rotation with a straight leg lying down on your back. Then, the toes point in toward the middle of your body. Lying on your stomach with your knee bent at 90 degrees, the toes point away (outward) from your body during internal rotation.

External rotation occurs when your feet roll out and toes point away from your body when lying on your back with legs straight out. This is the position many surgeons say needs to be avoided while recovering from hip arthroscopy to protect the hip joint capsule. If you are lying on your stomach with your knee bent at 90 degrees, external rotation occurs when the foot crosses the midline of the body toward the other side.

Flexion: A movement toward the front seen from the side. In terms of the hip joint, when you stand on two legs, then lift one leg up to a marching movement, flexion occurs at the hip joint. If you are lying down, the same applies. Sitting on a chair involves hip flexion. Bending your trunk forward also uses flexion in the hip. You can think of it as in being "in reverse." In both examples the angle between the thigh and the trunk decreases.

Extension: A movement toward the back, seen from the side, meaning that the angle of the front of the body increases. If you stand on both feet and move one leg back as if you are going to walk backwards or getting ready to kick a soccer ball, you are extending the leg. If you lie on your back and bring the leg back from flexion to a flat position on the bed, you are also extending the leg (back to the anatomically neutral position). *See Figure 9.*

These definitions and explanations just scrape the surface of all there is to know about movement. If you are interested in more in-depth reading about kinesiology, many good books are available. For the purposes of this book, being a practical patient guide, we are better off sticking to more basic explanations of movement. However, I want you to remember that physical therapists and other body workers think of movement in more complex terms than laypeople. Also, if like me, you want to be able to read and understand MRI reports and other medical reports, you may come across terms like "sagittal."

4.5 Muscle Agonists, Synergists and Antagonists

Muscles are so-called agonists, synergists and antagonists. Agonists are muscles that are primarily responsible for performing a specific movement. The word synergist indicates that muscles work in synergy, or together, to complete a task. Synergists are accessory muscles that assist agonists with a movement. The word antagonist indicates that a muscle works in opposition or against a different muscle, but that's not quite true. Instead, an antagonist works to control the rate and speed of a movement (8).

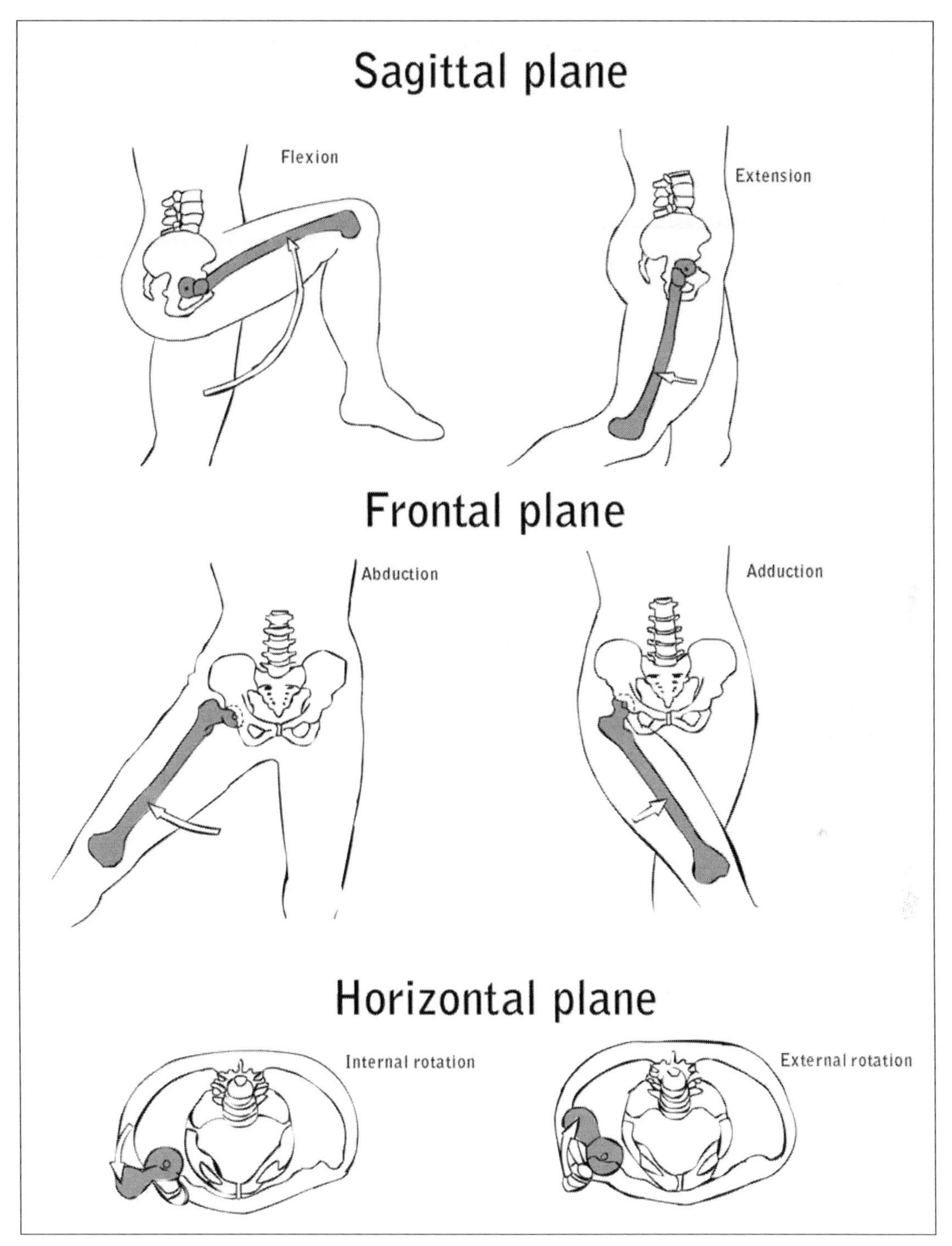

Figure 9: Femoral-On-Pelvic Hip Rotation

The illustration is modified from figure 12-23 in Donald A. Neumann's book *Kinesiology of the Musculoskeletal System*.

The concept of agonists, synergists and antagonists is best explained by an example:

Psoas is a primary hip flexor, an agonist. It receives help flexing the hip from, for example, rectus femoris and gracilis, which are synergists. Gluteus maximus (a primary hip extensor) is an antagonist in hip flexion and participates in the movement by providing resistance and helping to control the rate of the movement. If gluteus maximus weren't there to control the hip flexion, the leg would kick up uncontrollably. If a muscle that is supposed to be dominant in a movement is weakened, for a variety of reasons (a torn labrum possibly being one of them), other muscles that work together with the dominant muscle tend to get stronger than they should be. That is a type of muscle imbalance (8).

4.6 Bones of the Hip Joint and Pelvis

When we think about the hip joint, we may think of it as a pretty straight-forward ball-and-socket joint. As you might have guessed by now, it is much more complex than that. The socket portion of the hip joint actually is the union of three pelvic bones, called the ilium, ischium and pubis. This socket is in the pelvis. Together with the sacrum (the triangular-shaped bone at the lowest part of the spine), the ilium, ischium and the pubis form the bony pelvis. Rooted in Latin, the word pelvis means "basin" and is the lower portion of the trunk, bounded in the front and at the sides by the hip bones and in the back by the sacrum and tailbone (coccyx). *See Figure 10.*

The ilium is a fan-shaped bone and forms the upper part of the pelvis, to which are attached various muscles, including gluteal muscles, abdominals and spinal extensors. The upper rim of the ilium, which continues to the back of the pelvis, where it meets the sacrum, is called the iliac crest. Where the iliac crest ends, is often marked by dimples in the skin. At the front of the ilium are the two (one on each side) bony bumps that go by the medical term anterior superior iliac spine (ASIS). The bottom of the ilium holds the cup-shaped hip socket named the acetabulum (vinegar cup in Latin) (9).

The lower front part of the hip socket is where the hip meets the pubis. The pubic bones on each side create a joint — the pubic symphysis — in the middle of the body. A "spacer" made of fibrocartilage sits in the middle of that joint, and ligaments help hold it together. The ischium meets the hip joint in the lower rear part of the hip socket and goes from the rear of the pelvis, underneath to the pubis. *See Figure 11.*

Although the pubis and the ischium are considered separate bones of the pelvis, they are continuous bone structures without a dividing joint in adults. They are considered separate bones of the pelvis, because, prior to adulthood, they have a connection made of cartilage with clear boundaries, which turns into bone in the adult, making the boundaries less distinct. When you sit, you can feel what is commonly called the "sitting bones." The medical term is the ischial tuberosity, a part of the ischium. Many muscles attach here, for example the hamstrings and one of adductor magnus' two heads (9).

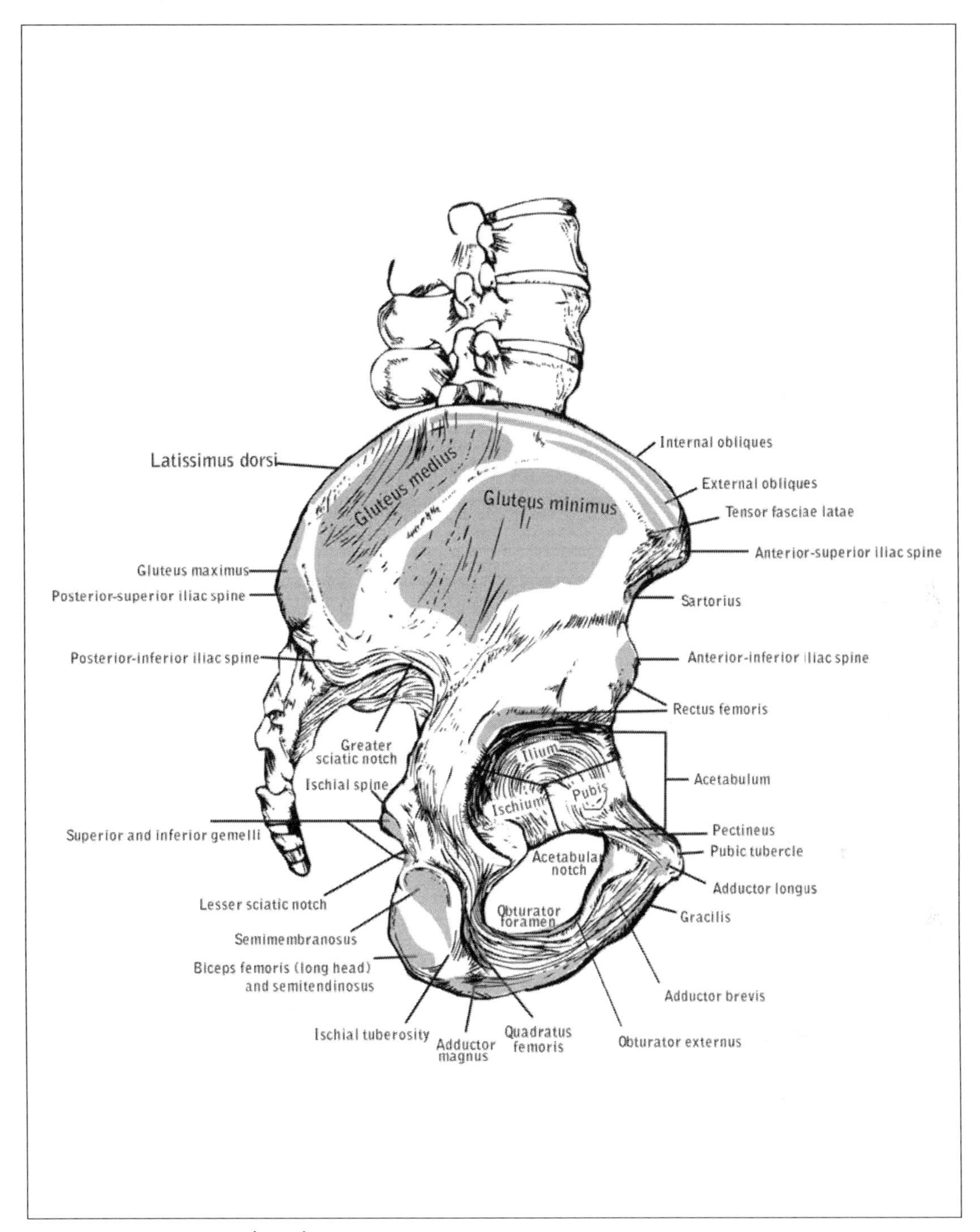

Figure 10: Lateral (side) view of the pelvis with a cross-section of the hip socket

The image shows the union of the ilium, pubis and ischium. Muscle attachments are shaded in grey.

The illustration is modified from figure 12-1 in Donald A. Neumann's book *Kinesiology of the Musculoskeletal System*.

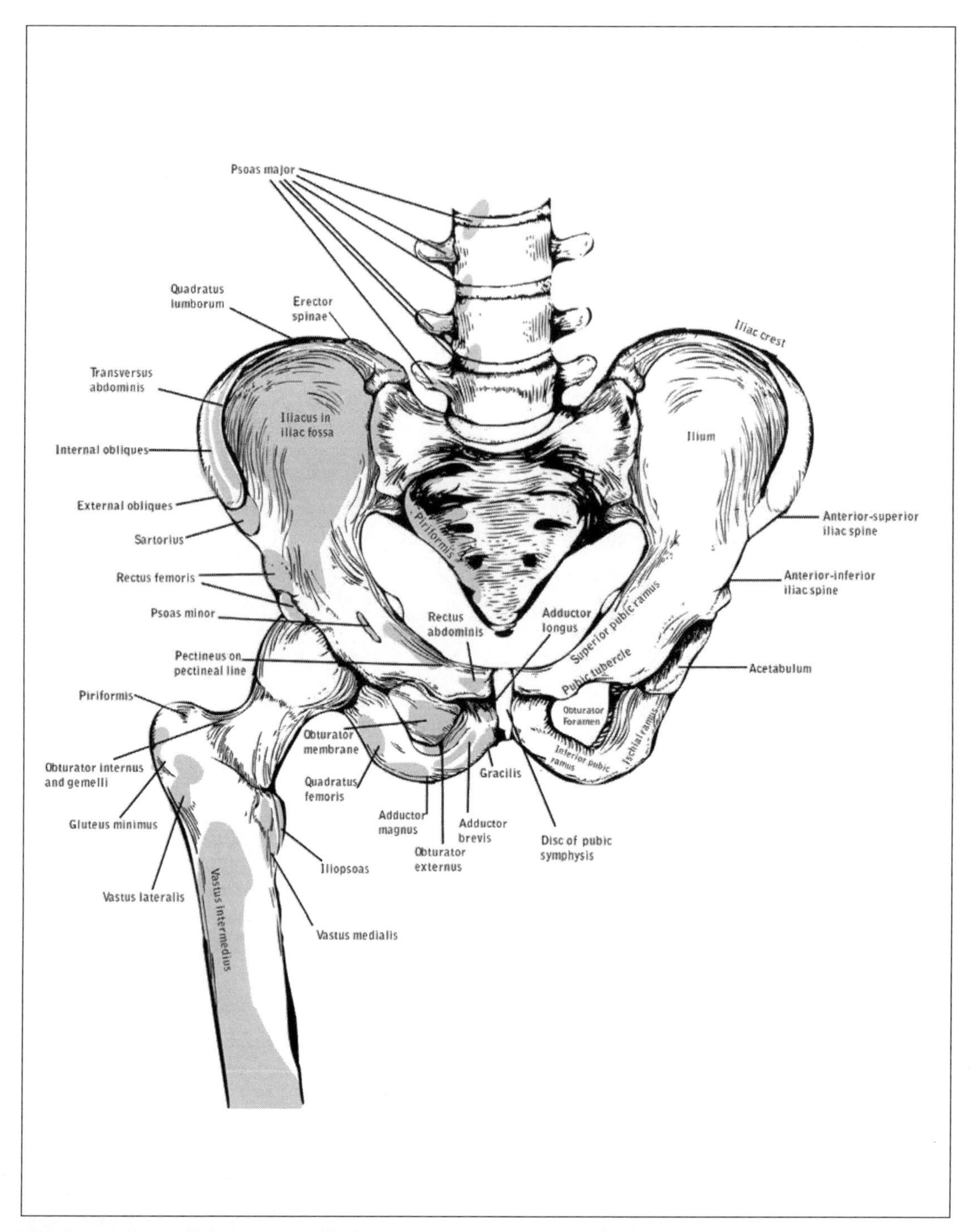

Figure 11: Anterior view of the pelvis, sacrum, and right upper femur

Muscle attachments shaded in grey.

The illustration is modified from figure 12-2 in Donald A. Neumann's book *Kinesiology of the Musculoskeletal System*.

Let's go back to the ilium, which holds the hip socket (acetabulum) and forms the upper part of the hip joint. The lower part of the hip joint is made up of the ball located on top of the thighbone. Femur is the medical term for thighbone. Consequently, the ball of the hip joint is called the femoral head. It rests on top of the femoral neck, which is a narrower part of the thighbone than the ball. The femoral neck is tilted on an angle from the femoral head, connecting the head with the thighbone. The femur's head is essentially round like a globe. But, as hip impingement patients are aware, there are anatomical variations. *See Figure 12.*

One thing to note about bone is that it conducts sound very well. Sometimes hip patients worry about clicking, popping and snapping. Because bone conducts sound and vibration readily, it is easy to assume that a snapping sound comes from the hip joint. However, there are plenty of other structures that can snap, especially tendons. The iliopsoas tendon runs right over the hip joint and is a frequent cause of snapping. The adductor longus tendon may click as can other tendons, too. Most often, popping sounds are of little significance, and, as muscles gain strength, snapping may subside. Clicking, snapping and popping are seldom a cause for worry (8).

4.7 Muscles of the Hip

Most of us who don't work in the medical field never have the opportunity to see the human body as it looks underneath the skin. Frankly, depending on your tolerance level to flesh, you may not want to. I myself am quite fascinated by the human body, so I made it to the exhibition "Bodies" in Las Vegas. I don't imagine it is quite like a cadaver dissection, but seeing the muscles, how they are layered, the muscle fibers, the innervation and the vascular system in 3-D reality offers you a whole new understanding of the human body — one that high school biology lessons or reading an anatomy book cannot equal. You will be much better off understanding some of the basics of anatomy and kinesiology. The more you know, the greater your advantage in talking to doctors, physical therapists and other medical professionals will be.

As you read the following subchapters on muscles, keep in mind that the muscles are stacked in layers. Between the muscles and even between individual muscle fibers there is fascia (connective tissue). In fact, fascia wraps just about everything in our bodies, down to the cells. Fascia is thin and whitish. Gross but true: Imagine trimming beef tenderloin. The thin whitish-transparent layer you trim away is fascia and looks much like human fascia. In its normal state, fascia is smooth and helps the layered muscles glide and function the way they are supposed to. The term fascia actually encompasses many kinds of related tissue. However, for the purposes of this book, I use the simplified description above.

When we are injured or muscles don't work properly, scar tissue or adhesions can form that impact the texture of the fascia: The fascia goes into a glue-like state. Rather than letting muscles glide against each other, they get stuck together by the fascial adhesions, making the muscles work improperly. In the chapter on rehabilitation, I will explore some options for

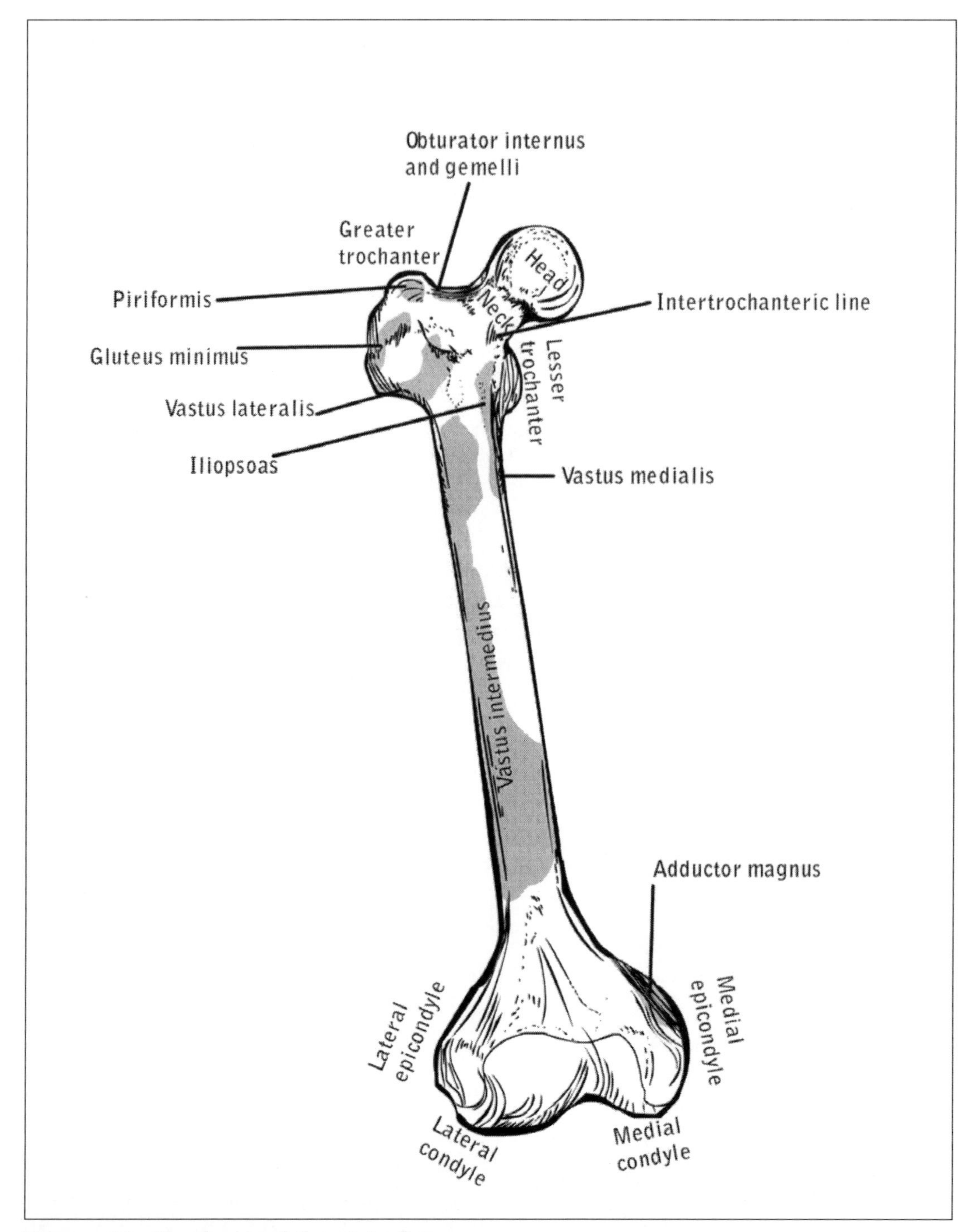

Figure 12: The front of the right femur

Muscle attachments are shaded in grey.

The illustration is modified from figure 12-4 in Donald A. Neumann's book *Kinesiology of the Musculoskeletal System.*

helping to break up adhesions. Unfortunately, some people are just more prone to making scar tissue and being fascially stuck. I'm not a researcher in scar tissue, but suspect the answer lies in the genetic makeup. For more information on fascia, Fascia: The Tensional Network of the Human Body by Robert Schleip (et al.) provides additional insight.

Looking at an anatomy chart, you will notice that the muscles of the hip joint have large areas of attachment, great length and large cross-sections (overlap). That makes them able to adapt their structure to a required function. Because of the way the hip muscles are aligned, and the great range of motion that is possible at the hip joint — picture the range of motion when doing a "split" in gymnastics —muscle functions are greatly influenced by the position of the hip joint. This means that muscles may perform one type of function when the hip is neutral, but a different function when the hip joint is flexed (10).

Now that I have explored some of the basic concepts that describe location and movement of muscles, as well as the layering of muscles and their ability to work in multiple ways, it is time to take a look at the actual muscle groups and individual muscles that provide motion to the hip joint. These are muscles that are often affected by hip impingement and the malfunctioning labrum. This book was written for patients and not for medical professionals, so the descriptions will be simplified and lack details that a medical professional would require. There is no lack of anatomy books for those who are hungry for more detailed information.

In the following subchapters, I will go over the muscle groups of the hip and the function of individual muscles. I am aware that muscles have specific origin and insertion points. For the purposes of this book, I decided to simply call them attachments.

4.7.1 Hip Adductors

As the name indicates, the primary function of the hip adductors is to adduct the hip — to bring the thigh toward the midline of the body. The adductors are a group of muscles consisting of adductor longus, adductor magnus, adductor brevis, pectineus and gracilis. There are also muscles that function as secondary hip adductors: Part of the biceps femoris (a hamstring), quadratus femoris (an external hip rotator) and the part of the gluteus maximus (a primary hip extensor). Simply explained, the adductors are located on the inside of the thigh. They lie in three layers, and attach close to each other along the pubic bone and further down on the thighbone along a ridge called the linea aspera. The exception is the gracilis muscle that attaches right below the knee on the inside of the lower leg.

Pectineus, adductor longus and gracilis are located in the top layer of adductors. Below them is a layer with one triangle-shaped muscle, the adductor brevis. The deepest layer of the adductors consists of only one large muscle, the adductor magnus. It has two so-called heads, one called the anterior head because it attaches on the front of the pelvis, and one called the posterior head that attaches on the ischial tuberosity ("sitting bones").

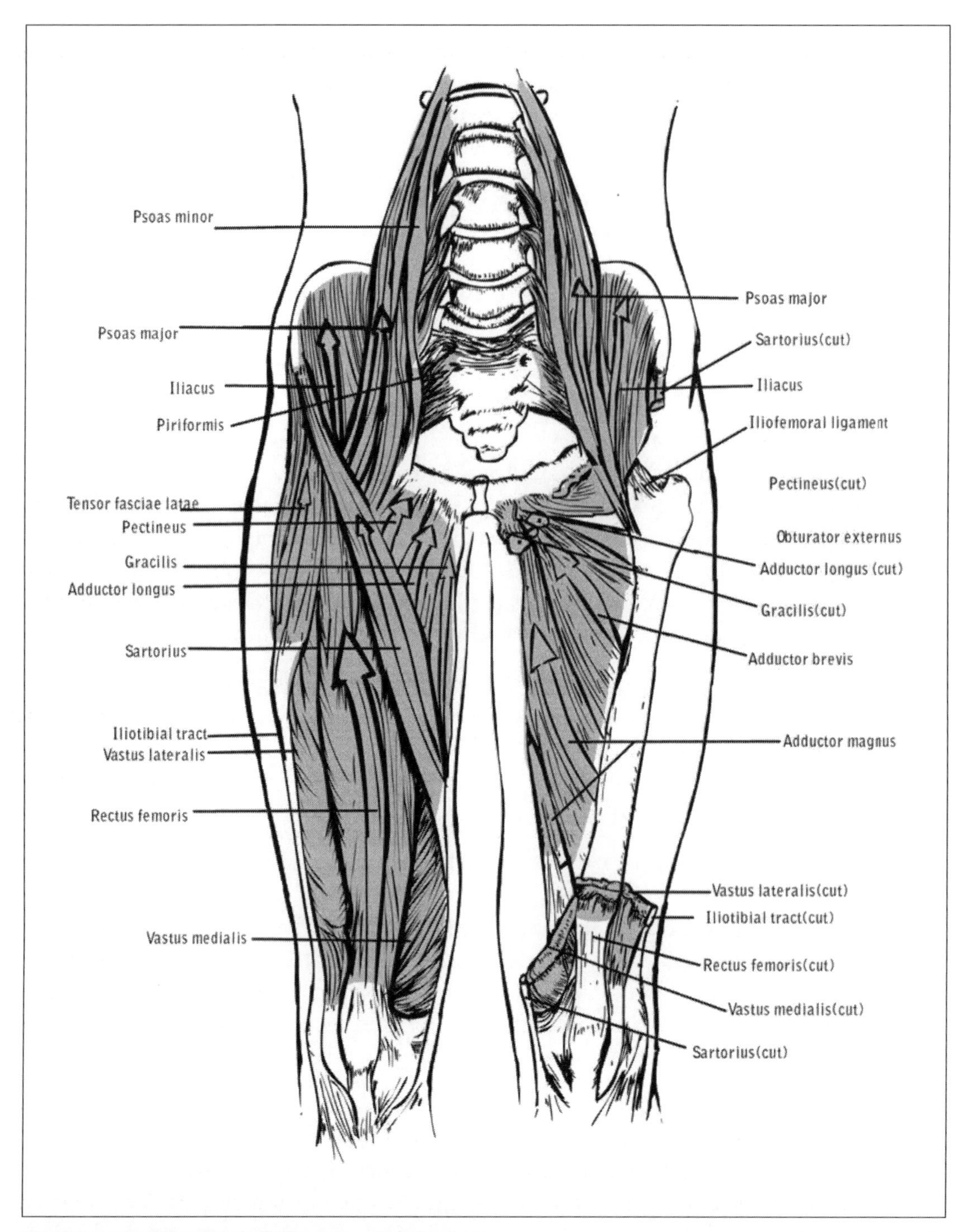

Figure 13: Muscles of the anterior hip

On the right, some muscles are cut to expose adductor brevis and adductor magnus.

The illustration is modified from figure 12-29 in Donald A. Neumann's book *Kinesiology of the Musculoskeletal System*.

Located right next to the hamstrings, part of the adductor magnus also functions as a hip extensor regardless of the position of the hip joint. Depending on the position of the hip joint, all the adductors except adductor magnus take on a secondary role as either hip flexors or extensors. When the hip joint is flexed at least 50-60 degrees during a fast sprint, the adductor longus, among others, provides the assisting capability of an extensor. When the hip is flexed less than 60 degrees, the adductor longus instead takes on the role of an augmenting hip flexor (9). *See Figure 13.*

The hip extension and flexion powers of, for example, adductor longus are very useful when you perform sports like sprinting, cycling and running up a steep hill, or coming up and down from a deep squat. The way we can put the adductors to use in multiple ways and directions also makes them quite susceptible to injury (9).

4.7.2 *Hip Abductors*

Abduction of the hip means moving the thigh away from the midline of the body. The primary hip abductors are the gluteus medius, gluteus minimus and tensor fasciae latae. The gluteus medius is by far the largest and the strongest of the abductors, providing about 60 percent of the hip the abduction force. It has one attachment on the ilium and another attachment on the outside of the thighbone, called the greater trochanter.

The gluteus minimus lies deeper than the gluteus medius, but also attaches on the ilium and on the greater trochanter. The tensor fasciae latae (TFL) is the smallest of the three primary hip abductors. It attaches on the outer surface (side) of the iliac crest and continues down on the side of the hip where it merges with the iliotibial band (IT band). The piriformis and sartorius are considered secondary hip abductors.

Abduction provides more than just movement to the hip. The abductors also work as important pelvis stabilizers during walking and produce joint force in the hip joint. When you take a step and swing one leg forward, the abductors in the leg that contacts the ground play an important role in controlling the pelvis. If the abductors weren't there to provide stability, the pelvis and the trunk would drop toward the side of the swinging leg. In that moment, the body's weight and the abductors are two opposing forces over the femoral head (ball of the hip joint) of the standing leg (9).

For every step you take, the pelvis is forced against the ball of the hip joint by the combined force created by the hip abductor muscles and the pull of body weight. To achieve linear balance, the force pressing down on the hip joint is counteracted by a joint reaction force of the same strength going in the opposite direction. The hip abductor muscles provide 66 percent of the forces that go into the hip joint (joint reaction force) (9). The hip abductors are essential to normal gait.

To give you a comparison: While only one leg is on the ground during walking, there is a hip joint reaction force of about 2.4 times the body weight. When you walk, but are not in the phase of single-stance (when one foot is on the ground), the force is even greater — about 2.5 to 3 times the body weight — due to accelerations of the pelvis. These forces increase to 5.5 times the body weight if you are running. Simple everyday activities such as getting up from a chair can actually produce joint pressures much higher than that. During sit-to-stand pressures on the hip socket reach 90 times the pressure in a full car tire (9).

The abductors are an important part of the stability of the pelvis and of the ability of the hip joint to counteract the forces placed on it. The cartilage in the hip joint protects the joint by dispersing these large forces as it provides a somewhat elastic, lubricated, and smooth surface. If you have arthritis in the hip, the cartilage of the hip may no longer be able to provide protection to the joint (9).

4.7.3 Hip Internal Rotators

Sometimes, the internal hip rotators are also called medial rotators. There aren't actually any primary internal hip rotators. This means that when the body is in its anatomic (anatomically neutral) position no muscles are optimally positioned to perform the internal rotation force. However, there are many secondary internal hip rotators. Depending on the position of the hip joint, different muscles contribute to internal rotation.

When the hip joint is flexed toward 90 degrees, part of the gluteus minimus and gluteus medius kick in to help with internal rotation of the hip. Several external rotators, for example the piriformis, switch their leverage and become internal rotators at 90 degrees hip flexion. When the hip joint flexes from 0 to 90 degrees, the internal rotation force dramatically increases for some of these muscles. That explains why the internal rotation force is about 50 percent greater with the hip flexed than with the hip extended. Many of the adductor muscles are also able to perform internal rotation of the hip when the body is in the anatomic position (9).

The internal rotators also fill an important function when you walk. While the left leg is on the ground (the stance phase) and the right leg is moving (the swing phase), the internal rotators twist the pelvis toward the left thighbone (stance leg). When the pelvis twists to the left you can see a forward rotation of the right ilium. In this example, the left internal rotator muscles actually give some of the drive to the right swinging leg (9).

4.7.4 Hip External Rotators

Sometimes, the external hip rotators are also called the lateral rotators. There are six short muscles included in the group of external hip rotators. Five of them can be categorized as the primary external rotators: piriformis, obturator internus, gemellus superior, gemellus inferior and obturator externus (the sixth one is quadratus femoris). In addition, the gluteus maximus and the sartorius muscles are considered primary external hip rotators. If you look at the pelvis from behind, the external rotator muscles lie horizontal, making them best suited to provide the external rotation force of the hip. They also help stabilize the back of the hip joint (9).

In very simple words, you can explain the location of the external hip rotators like this: They originate close to each other on the pelvis, on the bone called the ischium, around the area that most people would call the sitting bones, (except piriformis). They attach on the thighbone very close to the hip joint. The piriformis muscle originates on the inside (anterior) of the sacrum and goes to the outside of the thighbone. The sciatic nerve usually runs below the piriformis muscle. However, in some people, the sciatic nerve actually passes through the muscle belly of the piriformis muscle.

The obturator internus muscle takes a fascinating path. It arises from the inside of the obturator membrane, which is located right next to the "sitting bone" (ischial tuberosity). From there, the muscle fibers turn into a tendon which exits the pelvis while wrapping around the sciatic notch. The sciatic notch functions like a pulley and bends the tendon 130 degrees on its way toward the attachment on the thighbone, very close to the neck of the thighbone (9).

If you contract the left obturator internus muscle when the left thighbone is in a fixed position (during the stance phase of walking), the pelvis will rotate to the right. In this example the muscle works in reverse; it cannot rotate the hip as only the pelvis is free to move at this phase. The force produced by the left obturator internus compresses left the hip joint helping to stabilize it when the pelvis is rotated. The muscles called gemellus superior and gemellus inferior are located on either side of the obturator internus central tendon. They blend in with that tendon and attach together on the thighbone on the lower part of the neck below the ball of the hip joint (9).

The quadratus femoris is a flat muscle that goes from the outside of the "sitting bone" (the ischial tuberosity) and inserts on the back of the top of the thighbone. The obturator externus goes from the outside of the obturator membrane and attaches on the back of the thighbone. *See Figure 14.*

The functional potential of the external rotators is the most obvious during rotation of the pelvis on the thighbone. For example, the external rotators are hard at work when you abruptly change directions while running. If your right leg is firmly fixed on the ground, a contraction of the right external rotators (confusingly enough with more internal force than external force) moves the front side of the pelvis and the trunk away from the fixed thighbone. Now you can cut to the opposite side (9).

Muscles considered secondary external hip rotators include portions of the gluteus medius, gluteus minimus, biceps femoris and obturator externus (9).

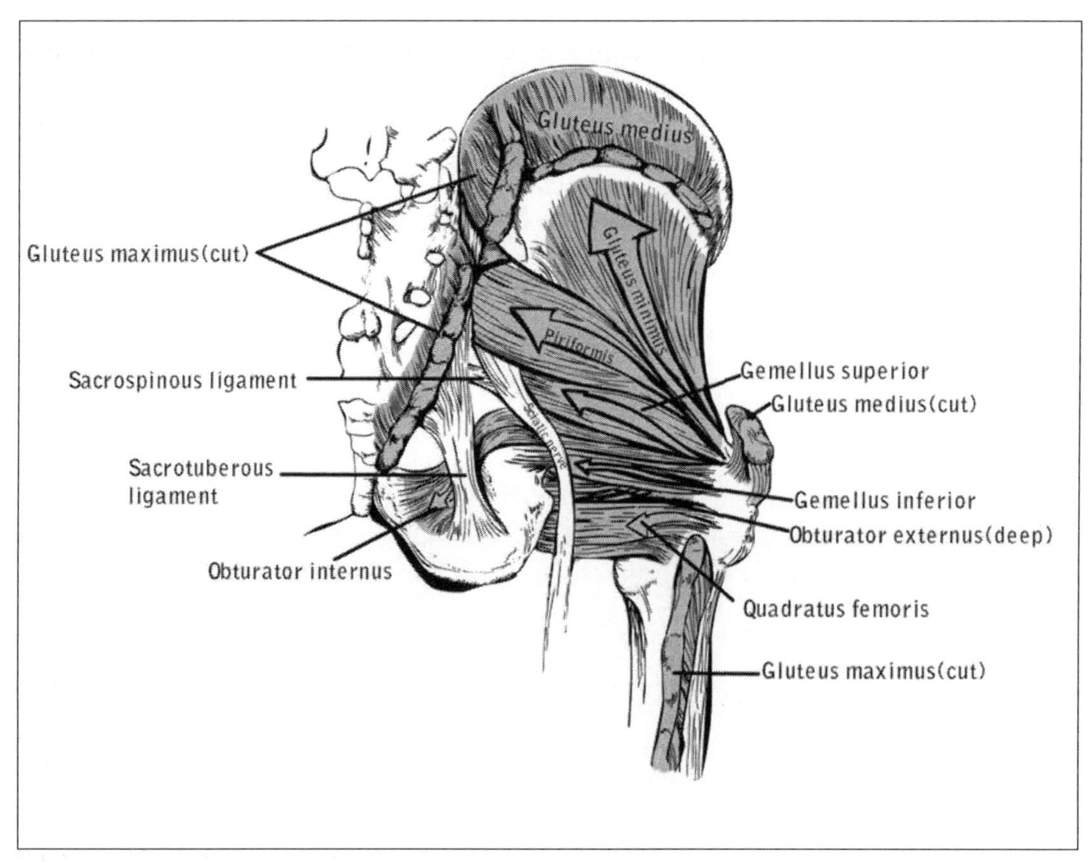

Figure 14: Muscles of the posterior and lateral hip

The gluteus medius and the gluteus maximus are cut to expose deeper muscles.

The illustration is modified from figure 12-44 in Donald A. Neumann's book *Kinesiology of the Musculoskeletal System.*

4.7.5 Hip Extensors

The primary hip extensor is the gluteus maximus, and the secondary is a muscle group called the hamstrings and a part of the adductor magnus. The hamstrings consist of biceps femoris, semitendinosus and the semimembranosus. Part of the gluteus medius works as a secondary hip extensor, and the adductor muscles can also extend the hip if the hip joint is flexed beyond 50 degrees.

The gluteus maximus, like the name suggests, is a large and powerful muscle that isn't only a primary hip extensor but also a primary hip external rotator. It has many attachments on the back of the pelvis and runs into the iliotibial band on the side of the thighbone as well as into the gluteal tuberosity which lies slightly behind the iliotibial band.

The hamstring muscles attach on the back of the sitting bone (ischial tuberosity) and extend to the lower leg bone, the tibia. They not only extend the hip, but also flex the knee, which is their primary function. As mentioned earlier (under Hip Adductors), part of the adductor magnus also functions as a hip extensor independent of the position of the hip joint. When the hip joint is flexed at least 50 to 60 degrees during a fast sprint, the adductor longus, among others, assists as a hip extensor. From a position of 75 degrees flexion at the hip joint, the hamstrings and adductor magnus produce an approximately equal amount of extension force — a total of 90 percent of the extension force possible at the hip. The remaining 10 percent is produced mostly by the gluteus maximus (9). The proportions change as the hip position approaches neutral.

The hip extensors also play a big role in helping to control a forward lean of the body, from something as simple as leaning forward to brush your teeth or to picking up a toy from the floor. The hamstrings carry the primary responsibility for this type of movement by limiting the degree of pelvic movement. The more you lean forward, the longer the hamstrings get, and the more they support the leaning position. In a different type of movement, if you imagine climbing a flight of stairs, the body mostly recruits the large gluteus maximus muscle instead to provide hip extension force (9). *See Figure 15.*

4.7.6 Hip Flexors

The hip flexors are often a trouble spot for hip impingement patients. The psoas (or iliopsoas) muscle is probably the best-known hip flexor, but there is a whole group of muscles called hip flexors. The primary hip flexors are iliopsoas, tensor fasciae latae, sartorius, rectus femoris, adductor longus and pectineus.

The psoas muscle is a large and long muscle that starts all the way up at the last vertebra of the thoracic spine (T-12), attaches along the lumbar spine and lies on the inside of the pelvis where it meets the iliacus muscle. Iliacus and psoas then exit the pelvis together, merge just in front of the hip joint before they wrap around the thighbone and form a tendon that attaches on the back of the thighbone below the hip joint. Because of how the psoas muscle is deflected and angled on its way through the body, it is a very strong hip flexor with a lot of force. When the hip is abducted, psoas can assist with external rotation. In addition to being a strong hip flexor, psoas is also a major stabilizer for the vertebraes of the lumbar spine (9).

Being the longest muscle in the whole body, sartorius has its own fame. If you put your fingers on the pelvis bones (anterior-superior iliac spine, ASIS) near the top of your front pant pockets, this is where your find the origination of sartorius. This very thin muscle crosses the front of the thigh diagonally and attaches below and on the inside of the knee. The root of the muscle's name is "sartor", which refers to a tailor's cross-legged seating position. That describes quite well all the functions this muscle is able to provide: hip flexion, external rotation and abduction (9).

The common working name for tensor fasciae latae is TFL. The short abbreviation is more indicative of its looks than its long Latin name. Indeed, TFL is quite short, attaches to bone on the ilium just to the side of sartorius and runs in to the iliotibial band (IT band) between

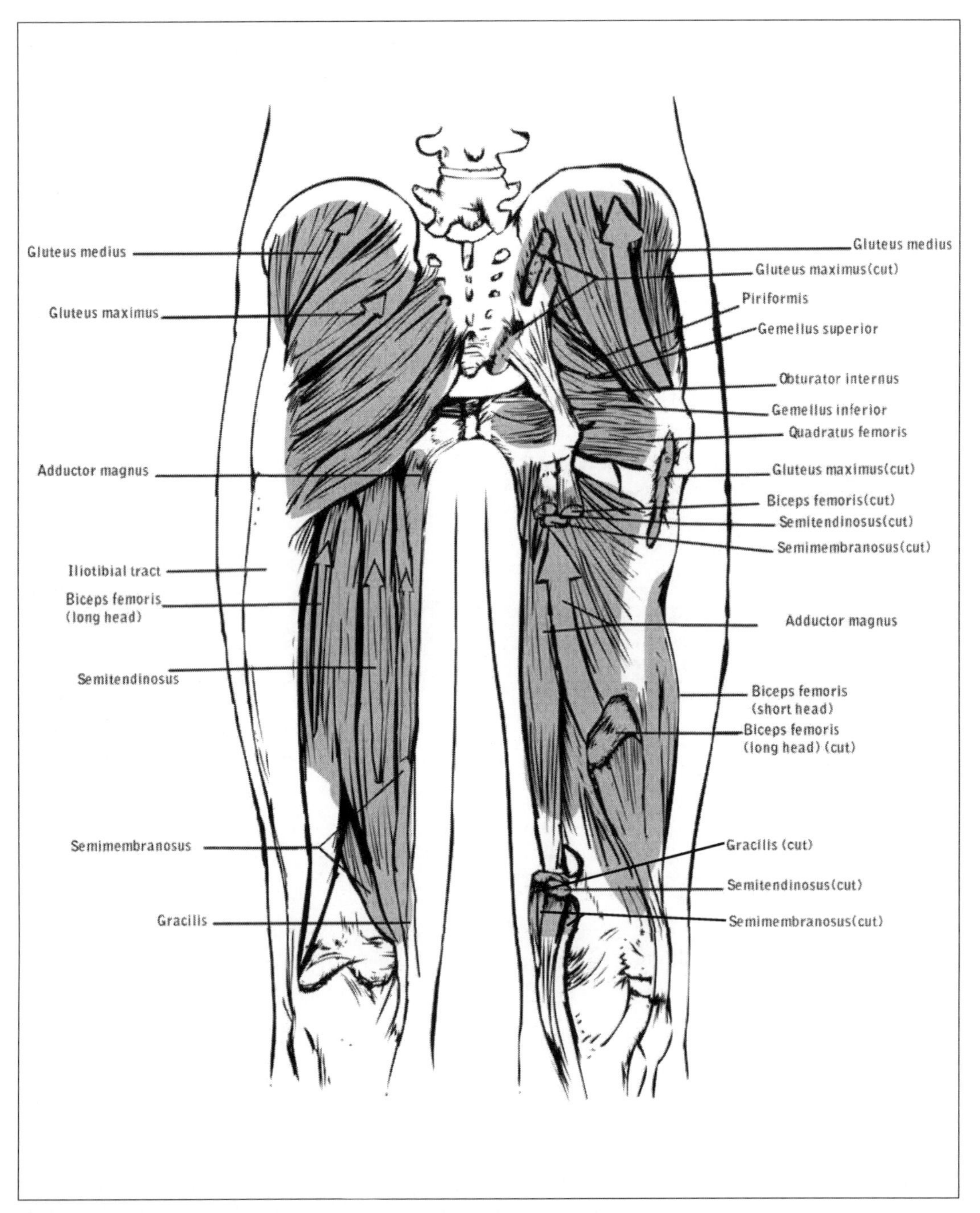

Figure 15: The posterior muscles of the hip

On the right, gluteus maximus and the hamstring muscles are cut to expose adductor magnus and the short head of biceps femoris.

The illustration is modified from figure 12-40 in Donald A. Neumann's book *Kinesiology of the Musculoskeletal System*.

the front and the side of the thigh. In its anatomic position, TFL is a primary hip flexor and abductor of the hip, but it can also work as a secondary internal hip rotator.

Rectus femoris is a large muscle and part of the group of muscles called quadriceps, or quads. It attaches close to sartorius at the ASIS along the top rim of the hip socket and into the capsule of the hip joint. Just like the other quads, rectus femoris extends downward and attaches to the bone in the lower leg, the tibia. This muscle provides about one third of the total isometric hip flexor force, but is also an important knee extensor (9).

In addition to being hip adductors, the adductor longus and pectineus also take on the role of primary hip flexors. When the hip is flexed less than 60 degrees, adductor longus helps with hip flexion. Muscles that are considered secondary hip flexors are adductor brevis, gracilis and part of the gluteus minimus. *See Figure 13.*

4.8 Nerve Supply to Hip Muscles and Hip Joint

Nerves from the lumbar spine (lumbar plexus) and the sacrum (sacral plexus) provide you with the ability to contract muscles surrounding the hip joint and to feel things in muscles and in the hip joint itself. In a simplistic way, a plexus can be described as a "box" where "cables" (nerves) enter and get mixed up before they split off again, as they exit the box. Motor nerves make it possible to control the contraction of a muscle. Sensory nerves receive stimuli (brain impulses) that enable you to notice how something feels. Nerves can have many different branches, and covering them all in detail would go beyond the scope in this book, but basic knowledge may help with your overall understanding of your specific situation and issues you may face.

Two major nerves than run from the lumbar plexus innervate the muscles of the front and the inside of the thigh: the femoral and obturator nerves. Nerves from the sacral plexus innervate the back and side of the hip as well as the back of the thigh and much of the lower leg. *See Figures 16 & 17*

4.8.1 *The Femoral Nerve*

The femoral nerve is the largest branch of the lumbar plexus. It provides motor branches to most hip flexors and all knee extensors. Inside the pelvis, the femoral nerve innervates the iliacus and psoas. It also sends branches to sartorius, part of pectineus and the quadriceps. This nerve also sends sensory branches to much of the skin of the front-to-middle part of the thigh. The hip capsule receives sensory innervation by the same nerve roots that supply the overlying muscle. Hence, the femoral nerve sends nerve threads into the front of the hip capsule. When doctors mention a small risk of nerve damage as a complication (see Possible Surgery Complications) from hip surgery, the femoral nerve is likely to be involved.

4.8.2 *The Obturator Nerve*

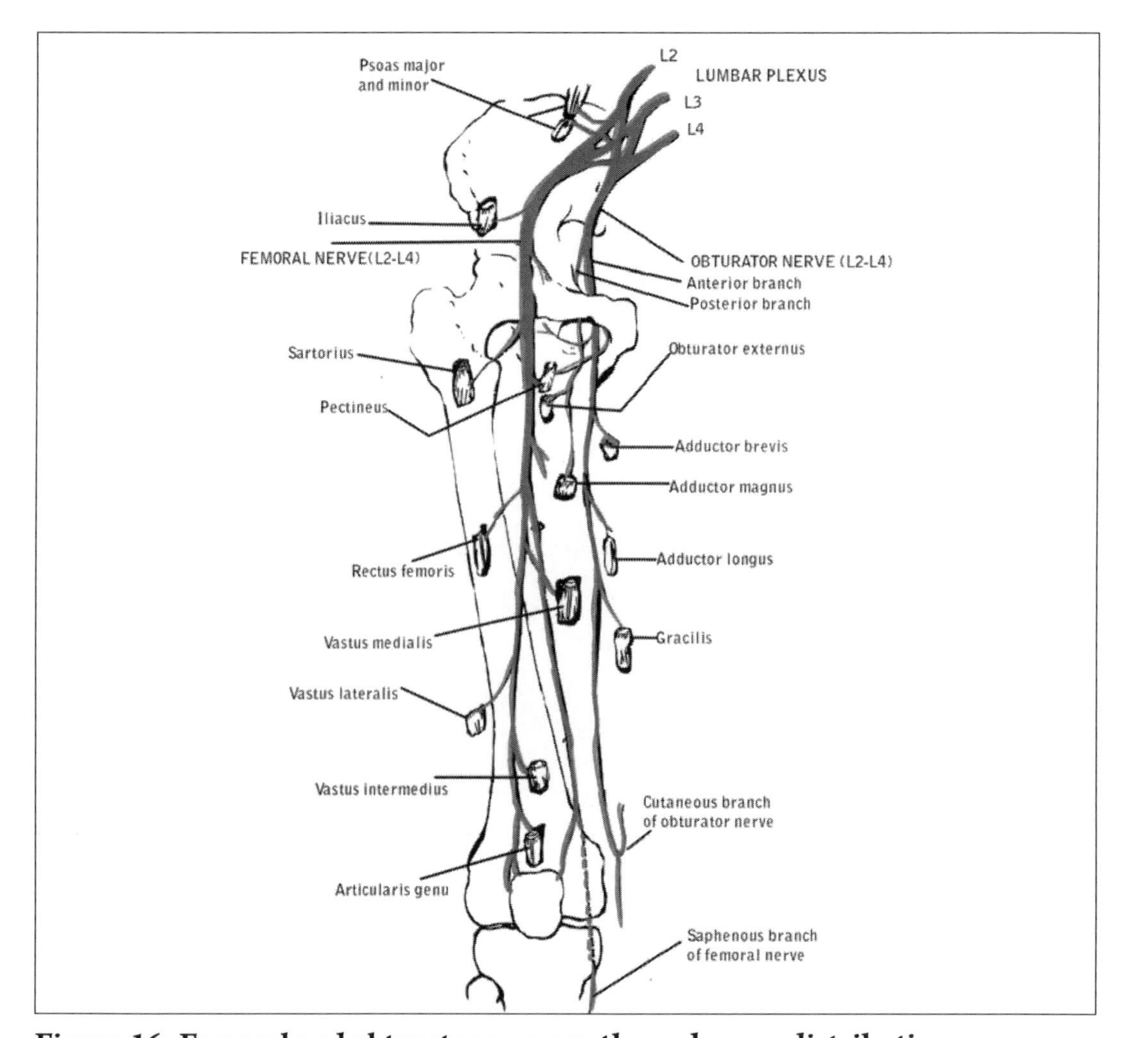

Figure 16: Femoral and obturator nerve paths and nerve distributions

The illustration is modified from figure 12-27 A in Donald A. Neumann's book *Kinesiology of the Musculoskeletal System.*

Just like the femoral nerve, the obturator nerve originates at the lumbar plexus. This nerve splits and sends motor branches both to the hip adductor muscles and to the hip rotator called obturator externus. The obturator nerve also provides skin sensation at the inside of the thigh. In the hip joint capsule, the obturator nerve sends threads to the medial hip capsule and to the knee joint. This explains why inflammation of the hip may be felt as referred pain in the knee toward the inside of the leg/knee (9). Sometimes, when hip patients complain about pain in the knee, and this pain is truly a referred pain, they have degenerative changes and arthritis, that is, inflammation, in the hip (6). Because of the complexity and spread of nerve pathways, a screening by a physical therapist of the whole region — foot to knee to hip to pelvis to lower thoracic spine — makes sense (8).

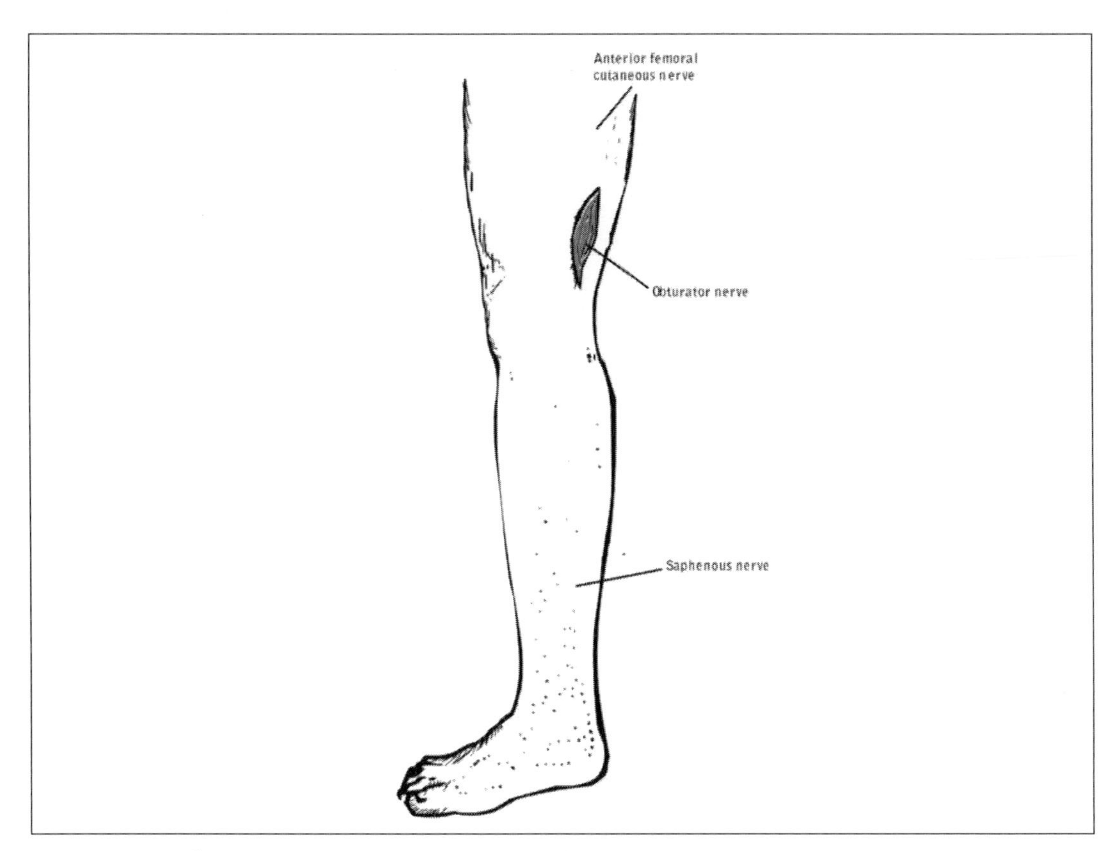

Figure 17: Thigh and leg nerve sensory distribution

The illustration is modified from figure 12-27 B in Donald A. Neumann's book *Kinesiology of the Musculoskeletal System.*

4.8.3 Nerves from the Sacral Plexus

Most nerves from the sacral plexus (L4-S4) send motor capability and sensation to the hip muscles in the back of the pelvis and the hip. The six short external hip rotators are innervated by small nerves that have uncreative names like "nerve to the piriformis." The gluteal muscles receive innervation by the superior and inferior gluteal nerves. The sciatic nerve is the widest and longest of the nerves from the sacral plexus. It is made up of two nerves, the tibial and peroneal nerves, enveloped by one connective tissue sheath. These nerves innervate the muscles in the back of the thigh. The tibial and peroneal nerves split at the knee; however, in some people the split occurs closer to the pelvis (9). In most people, the sciatic nerve exits the pelvis just under the piriformis muscle. However, in about 15 percent of people the sciatic nerve pierces the actual muscle belly of the piriformis, which may cause a condition called piriformis syndrome (7).

5 THE INCIDENCE OF HIP IMPINGEMENT

If you pulled a large number of random people off the street and performed imaging tests of their hips, you would find about a 15 percent incidence of hip impingement, more specifically CAM impingement. How do we know this? Because a study conducted by the Rothman Institute at Thomas Jefferson University Hospital, PA, did just that. Well, they didn't actually pull people off the street, but they used the CT scans of 419 randomly selected patients who were seen for conditions unrelated to their hips and who did not complain of hip pain.

The incidence of CAM impingement is about 15 percent of the population, but not everyone becomes symptomatic.

The study only looked for CAM impingement, which is easier to see on CT scans (and imaging in general) than pincer impingement. In measuring the α-angle on CT scans (see chapter 6.3.2.1 X-ray for explanation of α-angle) for the group of male participants, the study found 14 percent to 29 percent with abnormal angles. The number is a range because 15 percent had α-angles that were considered borderline abnormal. The equivalent result for the women was 5.5 percent to 6 percent (11).

Since the study didn't look for pincer impingement, it is easy to believe that the true incidence of hip impingement actually is greater than 15 percent of the population, especially since it is also possible that not all CAM lesions are detected by just measuring the α-angle (11).

Some researchers have suggested that there is a radiological blind zone at the front-to-side quadrant of the thighbone head-neck junction. They say that if there is not a bump at this spherical junction doctors would miss seeing CAM lesions and underestimate an FAI deformity (12). Taking those findings into consideration, the actual incidence of CAM impingement could be even greater than 15 percent.

5.1 Athletics or Genetics?

If the topic of hip impingement is not new to you, you have probably come across this question before: Is hip impingement caused by genetic factors or by an athletic lifestyle? The answer and literature, so far, is inconclusive. There is no simple yes-or-no answer.

If you have hip impingement, but have never jogged, skated or kicked a soccer ball in your life, I am sure you would be inclined to say that FAI is caused by genetics. But the fact is that physicians still don't understand the exact cause of hip impingement. Many physicians currently believe that hip impingement is a condition caused by a combination of athletics and genetics. At this point, there is no systematic approach to consistently identify persons at risk of developing hip impingement ahead of time. "If everyone lived under water [because water decreases joint impact] and had a sedentary job, would the incidences of FAI go down dramatically? Potentially. We certainly see it more often in active individuals that require more aggressive motion of the hip." (6)

If, like me, you have tirelessly scouted the Internet for articles, blogs etc. on hip impingement you might have read theories about how athletics in your youth, before all joints have finished growing, can cause hip impingement. According to FAI specialist Dr. Chad Hanson, there is no research to back such statements. He does note, however, that kids who suffer a slipped capital femoral epiphysis (SCFE, a separation of the ball of the hip joint from the thighbone at the upper growth plate of the bone) tend to have big CAM-like lesions. Other children who have a condition called Perthes Disease can also have an abnormal shape of the acetabulum (hip socket). "So, certainly growth is an important component to the anatomy that we see in femoroacetabular impingement, but there is no conclusive research to support the assertion that athletics before your bones are fully developed is the main contributing factor for FAI" (6).

Considering one fairly large study suggested that at least 15 percent of the general population have CAM lesions, but far from all are symptomatic (although it doesn't mean that they couldn't become symptomatic), it seems unlikely that genetics is the only component of FAI-induced pain. As time goes by, physicians become more familiar with FAI, and studies can follow participants over a longer period of time, maybe we will get a better answer as to what causes FAI.

6 DIAGNOSING HIP IMPINGEMENT

Receiving a correct diagnosis of hip impingement and labral tears isn't always easy. When I saw my hip surgeon for the first time, I felt like I had to present a case to him along the lines of "I know there is something wrong with me. I think I have this. Please help me!" My slightly desperate approach was not a consequence of how that doctor treated me, but caused by all of the other doctors I had seen before him who never helped me.

The doctor then told me, that the odds of getting a correct diagnosis were now clearly in my favor. This gave me some comfort. Having seen so many medical providers that I had lost count, and spent so many years trying to figure it out, I learned that while I was a statistical average-bumper, I was certainly not an anomaly — at least not according to a 2006 study in the *Journal of Bone and Joint Surgery*. That study looked at the mean time from onset of symptoms to the diagnosis of a labral tear and concluded that it took the average patient 21 months and a mean of 3.3 health care providers to receive a correct diagnosis for a labral tear (13).

I learned that while I was a statistical average-bumper, I was certainly not an anomaly.

Sometimes, depending on the degree and type of impingement, getting diagnosed with FAI is rather straightforward. Sometimes, it takes quite a few diagnostic steps and specialized expertise. At the physical therapist's office, I've had the pleasure of chatting with some hip patients younger than me, in their teens or twenties. Getting correctly diagnosed the first time you show up at a doctor's office is being privileged in terms of FAI. I envy those of you who do. In the following chapter, I will cover the FAI symptoms, how to find the right doctor to diagnose you, and what the diagnostic steps entail.

6.1 Hip Impingement Symptoms

The most common complaint among patients with hip impingement is pain of some sort. A large study from 2007, conducted by Dr. Philippon (and others), followed patients from the time they were first seen at the Steadman Clinic in Vail, Co., a large center for arthroscopic hip surgery, through receiving a diagnosis of FAI, until well after the surgery. Three-hundred and one hip arthroscopies performed to treat FAI, labral tears and cartilage defects were included in the study. Eighty-five percent of patients complained about moderate or marked pain — pain severe enough to seek treatment. Anterior groin pain was the most common complaint and occurred in 81 percent of patients. Of the 301 patients all but one, that is, 300 patients or 99 percent were found to have associated labral tears; 82 percent of the patients also had other cartilage defects (3). My surgeon once told me that my problems with pain probably didn't escalate until I tore my labrum. If you read about the function of the labrum earlier, it is evident how a malfunctioning labrum can contribute to developing muscle imbalances, secondary injuries and pain.

According to the above study, sometimes the pain can be located on the side of the hip (over the greater trochanter) or in the buttock region. The study also reported that, although groin pain is the most common complaint amongst FAI patients, there is a significant overlap with other regions of pain; 61 percent of the patients expressed having pain on the side of the hip; 52 percent complained of deep buttock pain; 23 percent reported sacroiliac joint pain (3).

The pain caused by FAI may be a consistent dull ache and/or catching and popping. Pain is often triggered by simple activities like getting in and out of a car, getting up from a seated position after a long time, or any type of rotation that involves a lot of bending of the hip (6). The 2007 study also noted that stiffness that greatly limited activity was a complaint among a third of all patients. Thirty-four percent of the patients reported feeling weakness that limited their activity (3).

Sometimes patients experience popping and snapping that is not actually inside the hip joint. For example, the psoas muscle or rectus femoris (both primary hip flexor muscles) can snap or crunch. It is still up for debate whether labral tears themselves actually cause clicking sounds, although some researchers suggest that this is the case. No matter the source of the clicking or snapping, 25 percent of the participating study patients reported that such clicking and snapping limited their activity to a great extent. In addition, feelings of instability or giving way were reported by 26 percent of the patients (3).

The pain caused by FAI may be a consistent dull ache and/or catching and popping.

Diagnosing FAI can be challenging because the symptoms do not always present as clear-cut hip problems. Due to the complex nature of the pelvis and the hips, many differential diagnoses can be made. Sometimes, such diagnoses are made even though the patient has hip impingement, and the impingement is the source of the pain. Several studies that included patients who were eventually treated for FAI, reported that patients had been either offered and/or received treatment for a variety of conditions — treatments that failed to resolve the pain. These differential diagnoses and procedures included knee arthroscopy, lumbar discectomy, ovarian cyst laparoscopy, iliotibial band or trochanteric bursitis procedures, hernia exploration and psoas or tendon releases (3).

Because no one wants to have unnecessary surgery, and the FAI symptoms of groin pain, side hip pain and buttock pain are quite unspecific and can involve many different conditions, it's crucial to get the right diagnosis and identify when hip impingement is the source of the pain. On the other side of the coin, sometimes there isn't just THE pain but several kinds of pain, potentially from multiple sources. You can have symptoms that fit with FAI, have FAI, and also have other sources of pain that aren't directly produced by the hips. Those symptoms could be injuries secondary to FAI (like athletic pubalgia or "sports hernia") or a completely separate issue (like uterine fibroids causing groin pain).

It may even take fixing one source of pain, like FAI, to be able to distinguish one pain from the other then and move on to fixing remaining issues. Even if you have FAI, and clearly have problems related to labral tears, not all of your groin pain need necessarily be a direct referred pain from the hip joint. Adductor pain from overuse or injury, for example, can be a major source of groin pain that is caused by, but not directly referred from, the hip joint.

Sacroiliac pain and knee pain can be seen in patients with hip impingement. Such symptoms can be confusing because they would not immediately lead a physician who is not an FAI specialist to think of the hips as the source of the pain. Many hip patients have had lumbar spine MRIs and physical therapy to treat what is perceived as a back pain issue. In my case, buttock pain led doctors to send me out for lumbar and pelvic MRIs. Unfortunately, there is a high incidence of false-positive lumbar spine MRIs that may send patients in the wrong direction when it comes to getting a diagnosis of FAI. Numerous studies have included MRIs for patients who did not have lower pain back and showed varying degrees of false-positive lumbar spine MRIs. The average result of the studies indicated that 38 percent of MRIs show a disc bulge without causing any symptoms of a disc bulge. The equivalent average for disc protrusions was 29 percent (14).

Sacroiliac pain and knee pain can be seen in patients with hip impingement.

If your pain patterns are complex, you can see how important it is to have skilled doctors who, in addition to mastering their specialties, also take a very systematic approach to diagnosis.

6.2 Finding the Right Doctor

Reading this book you might already suspect that you have hip impingement, but may not have found anyone to make that diagnosis for you, or you may have received a diagnosis and are looking for a surgeon to trust. An FAI surgeon can probably perform other types of orthopedic surgeries (ACL surgeries of the knee are pretty standardized these days), but that doesn't mean that any orthopedic surgeon can successfully perform an FAI surgery and give you a lasting good outcome.

Sometimes, where you live and the type of insurance coverage you have may put obstacles in your way. But please don't let that stop you from finding the right doctor. It is crucial to find an FAI surgeon who gets it right the first time, because nobody wants to go through revision surgery. If you have read my story, it will be clear to you that finding the right doctor to diagnose and treat FAI was half of my struggle. There is not an abundance of doctors with right expertise to make the correct diagnosis, choose the right treatment and perform the 'eries with excellence. In the following section, I will review what you can do to find out if .. uoctor is truly an FAI specialist and not a just an orthopedic surgeon who claims to do hips.

6.2.1 *Who is Who in Hip Arthroscopy?*

Regrettably, there are surgeons who market themselves as hip specialists or hip arthroscopists and as competent in performing FAI surgery who don't really fulfill those criteria. When you evaluate if a doctor fits your needs, it is helpful to find out where and under whom s/he trained, and to get a good idea of what the surgeon's (arthroscopic) FAI treatment philosophy is. Someone who claims to do FAI surgeries should be able to elaborate on the procedure. So let him or her do just that. You are interviewing someone to do a very important job for you. Ask open-ended questions to allow the doctor to show his or her competence or lack thereof. The answers to such questions will give you a good idea of what the surgeon's goal is with the surgery. Of course, to do so, first, you need to be an informed patient.

Examples of questions you may want to ask a surgeon are:

What is your philosophy on hip arthroscopy? What do you do once you are inside the joint?

How do you make sure to you don't shave too little or too much bone?

What is your approach to a torn labrum — repair or debridement?

When is microfracture a warranted procedure? What is your experience with microfracture?

How much joint space do you require the patient to have to perform hip arthroscopy?

What measures do you take to protect the joint capsule?

What is your protocol for post-surgical physical therapy?

What restrictions do you ask your patients to follow after surgery, during the recovery phase?

What was your training in FAI surgery?

Who did you train under and where?

You should expect that a skilled FAI surgeon reads your imaging films him/herself. The physician should correlate the physical exam findings to the images and explain them to you. An FAI surgeon should not put blind faith in a written radiology report and just treat according to that report. A surgeon who shows you your bone deformities, tears and dysfunction will help you understand the process of getting better.

If you get the feeling that the surgeon is more interested in getting into the joint, getting a good visual of it, diagnosing and doing a little bit of treatment that is probably not enough for a good outcome. Let the surgeon prove to you that s/he is competent in altering the biomechanics of the joint, changing the junction at the head and neck of the thighbone, shaving the bone down to a more anatomic shape, repairing and reattaching the labrum and getting better long-term functional results (6).

If you live in a rural area you are probably used to traveling for medical care. Some states don't have a single FAI-specialized doctor. That makes it challenging to find the right doctor, and even more important to do plenty of research before spending the time and money to go see a specialist far away. If you do live far from an FAI specialist, it may be possible to send medical records, imaging etc. to him or her for an evaluation and have a short phone consult to see if the trip is worth it. Big city folks can start by inquiring at a research hospital in the orthopedic clinic for an orthopedic physician with specialized training in FAI arthroscopic hip surgery. Fortunately, the understanding of hip impingement is increasing and so is the number of specialists. At least, you can expect to find greater understanding and expertise now than 10 years or even 5 years ago. There are several groups dedicated to FAI on Facebook; there you can connect with other FAI patients and get help finding names of surgeons.

Fortunately, the understanding of hip impingement is increasing and so is the number of specialists.

When you interview surgeons to perform FAI surgery, it may be helpful to find out who the surgeon's mentor is. "Who your mentor is shapes how you approach the hip. Everyone has their own approach to the way they get into the hip, how aggressive they are with the labrum, the bone resection and the physical therapy afterwards." (6)

Some of the best-known hip arthroscopists and mentors of many other FAI surgeons are Dr. Marc J. Philippon, Dr. Thomas Byrd and Dr. Thomas Sampson.

Dr. Marc J. Philippon at the Steadman Clinic in Vail, Co., is one of the world's most renowned surgeons for arthroscopic surgery of the hip. He has developed many of the joint preserving arthroscopic techniques used today, and continues to be an active researcher. The Steadman Clinic offers a fellowship program for orthopedic surgeons to receive specialized training in arthroscopic procedures of the hip, knee and shoulder. You can find more information including bios of all the physicians that have completed the fellowship program at: http://thesteadmanclinic.com.

In Tennessee, there is a physician named Dr. Thomas Byrd, who is also a pioneer in developing the art of hip arthroscopy. Dr. Byrd is also an active researcher who continues to evolve the area of hip arthroscopy. Dr. Byrd works out of Nashville Sports Medicine and Orthopaedic Center. More info can be found at http://www.nsmoc.com/.

Another well-known name in FAI and hip arthroscopy circles can be found outside of San Francisco. At Post Street Surgery Center, Dr. Thomas Sampson sees patients for hip impingement. You can find more information on Dr. Sampson at http://www.poststreetsurgery.com.

When finding a surgeon to evaluate you and possibly perform surgery, I realize that most of us have limitations like a geographic area, insurance network and finances. If one of the big names is not an option for you, there are definitely other great options. These specialists train other physicians. So, one way you can go about finding an FAI specialist is to inquire with their offices or research their websites for where in the country FAI doctors they trained are now in practice.

As is common in the field of medicine, you will find that doctors have differing opinions or even opposing views on arthroscopic hip surgery, diagnostic methods and rehabilitation after surgery. In reviewing the websites of the three surgeons mentioned above, I found that all three claim to have pioneered the area of arthroscopic hip surgery or even invented the method.

So who is right and who is wrong? For you, as a patient, it doesn't matter all that much who claims the prize. What matters is understanding that there are variances in how doctors do surgery and what type of post-surgical rehabilitation they propose. In some areas, opinions may vary greatly.

As patients, we need to understand that hip arthroscopy is still in evolution.

Physical therapy after surgery is one such area of disagreement. Some specialists may recommend early and aggressive physical therapy to restore range of motion and potentially reduce adhesion formation. Others may have a respite period to allow for healing before moving forward with therapeutic intervention. This aspect of the treatment of FAI continues to evolve (6).

Dr. Hanson points out that during the past three to five years much in terms of hip arthroscopy has been standardized, but the techniques continue to evolve, as surgeons strive toward finding better, easier and more reproducible surgical techniques. Without computer-navigated osteoplasty to reliably and consistently remove bone lesions in the hip, hip arthroscopy remains very much an art, and is not always performed reliably across the country (6).

As patients, we need to understand that hip arthroscopy is still in evolution. The technology, surgical equipment and physicians' understanding of the anatomy, and the joint positioning is all improving. The goal of physicians over the last several years has been to convert FAI surgery from an art to a science. When doctors can create objective criteria for how much bone to shave and how aggressive to be with the labrum, FAI surgery will become standardized. This will make it easier for surgeons across the country to implement it with good outcomes. The situation can be compared to the early days of ACL reconstruction in the knee joint. Now, many orthopedic surgeons know how to do successful ACL reconstructions. There are far fewer surgeons who are very comfortable with hip arthroscopy.

If hip arthroscopy is an art, I'd like my artist to be a masterful painter — really steady on the brush — because the canvas he's painting on is me.

6.3 Steps to Diagnosing Hip Impingement

Now that I have explored some of the key issues in identifying a specialized FAI surgeon, it is time to review the steps for correctly diagnosing FAI. When you meet with an FAI specialist for an evaluation, he or she should always take a detailed history from you, and get a good sense of your feeling of what precipitates the hip pain and where the pain is located. You should expect a thorough exam and various impingement tests. Imaging will be a natural part of obtaining more data about your hip joints. Depending on the findings and your medical history, a course of conservative treatment may be the right choice, or advanced imaging and diagnostic injections may be performed.

6.3.1 Pain Tests

How skilled the doctor is at performing so-called pain tests and at reading imaging may be crucial to your diagnosis. As a patient, it is important to know what to look for during your initial visit, and be informed of the specific testing for FAI to get a feel for the surgeon's specialization.

6.3.1.1 The Anterior Impingement Test

Anterior is medical speak for something as simple as front or in front of. The early literature on FAI and labral tears spoke of anterior impingement. Today, that term is not as commonly used to describe disease in the hip. However, the anterior impingement test does test for CAM impingement and labral tears in the front of the joint, which is the most accessible with arthroscopic instruments. The keywords for the anterior impingement test are flexion, adduction and internal rotation (FADIR). When your doctor performs this test, you will be lying down on your back on an examination table. He or she will flex your hip to 90 degrees, then adduct the leg (move your leg inward to the middle of your body and beyond if possible) and at the same time internally rotate your leg (ankle points out and knee points in).

Dr. Chad Hanson describes the anterior impingement test: "If you imagine a child going into a sitting 'W-position,' which we should not ever encourage them to do, you are recreating that position. In patients with FAI, the anterior impingement test drives the CAM lesion into their chondrolabral junction [the contact area between joint cartilage and labrum]" (6). According to the large study (referenced in the chapter on Hip Impingement Symptoms) performed in 2007 at the Steadman Clinic, the anterior impingement test was positive, that is, it reproduced pain, in 99 percent of the patients who had FAI (3). With that in mind, I dare say that a correctly performed anterior impingement test is an essential part of the diagnostic puzzle for FAI. *See Figure 18.*

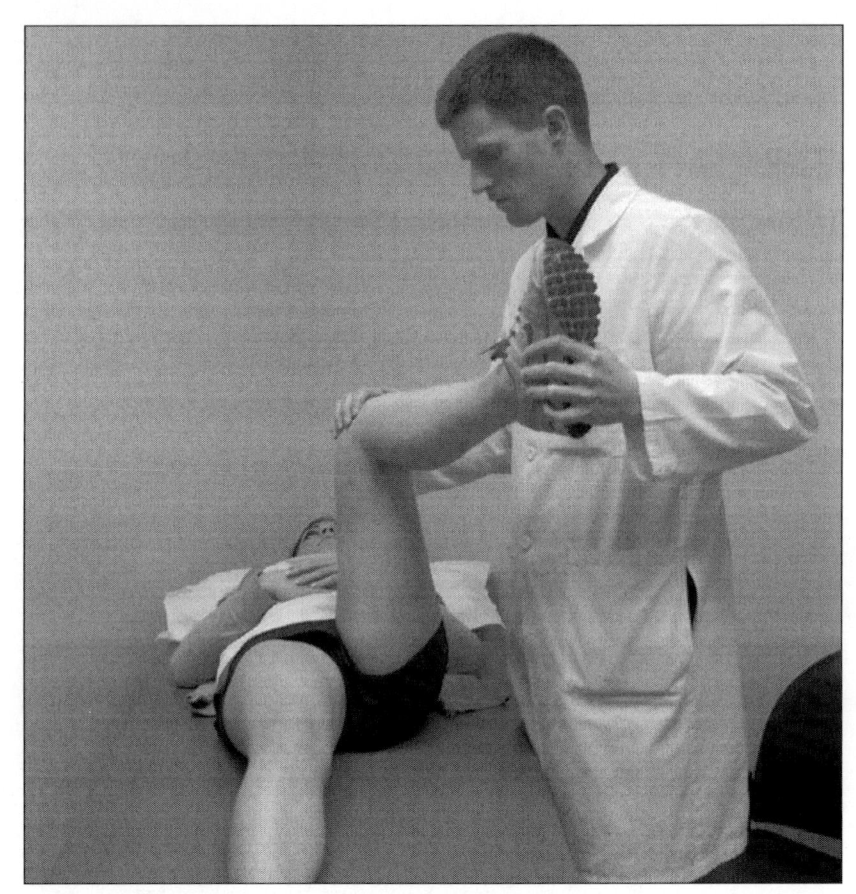

Figure 18: The anterior impingement test
Photography by Jeffery Newburn.

6.3.1.2 Posterior Impingement Test

If you didn't already know, by now you have probably gathered that posterior means back, in the back or behind. Does that mean that there is such pathology as posterior impingement? Logically, one would think so, but no. The posterior impingement test provides another way to test for labral pathology. Not every patient feels pain in the front of the hip/thigh. Sometimes patients don't have pain with the anterior impingement test, but they do with the posterior test. Consequently, in order not to let impingement go undiagnosed, your doctor should evaluate using both the anterior and posterior impingement tests (6).

Sometimes confused with each other, the posterior impingement test and the FABER test are not the same test. The posterior impingement test entails leg extension and external rotation, usually at end of an examination table. You will be lying down on your back with your bottom scooted all the way to the edge of the examination table. With your legs stretched out (extended) and hanging off the end of the table, the tester will hold one leg and externally rotate it so that the toes point either to the left (for the left leg) or to the right (for the right leg). If

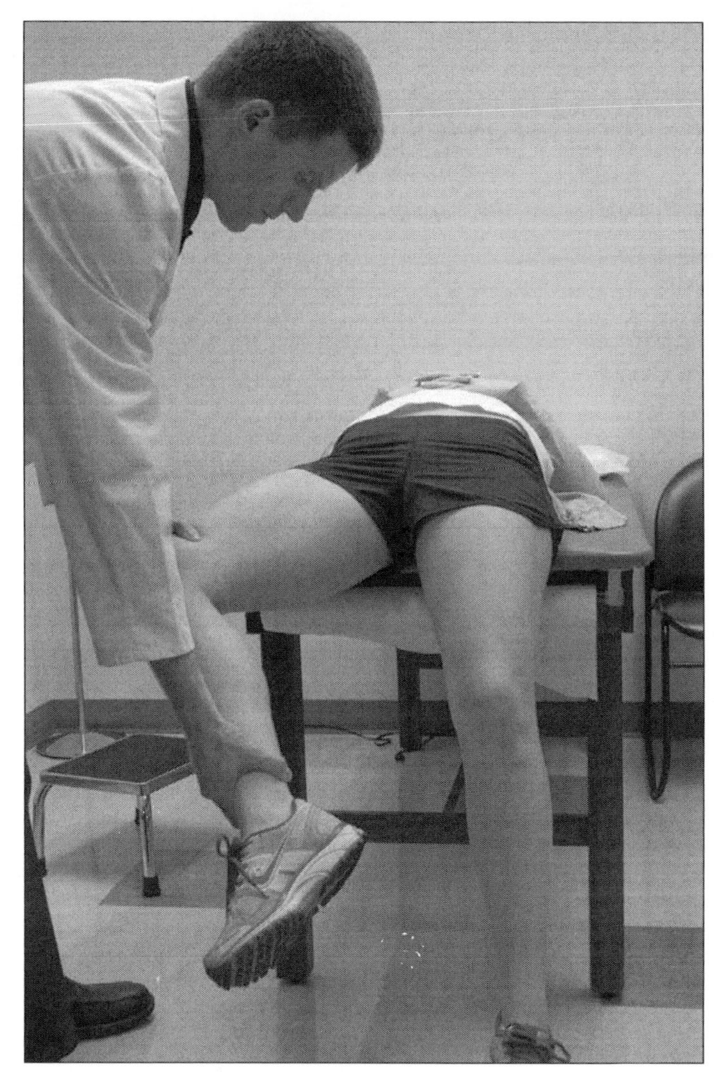

Figure 19: The posterior impingement test
Photography by Jeffery Newburn.

there is pain or restriction at the hip joint in this position, it may give a clue about whether labral tears, impingement, or instability may be present (6). *See Figure 19.*

6.3.1.3 FABER Test

Your doctor might also do a FABER (flexion, abduction and external rotation) test. During the FABER test, you will be lying on your back on the examination table. With gentle force the doctor will place your foot on the opposite knee and then rotate the knee to where it is essentially flat down on the table while stabilizing the opposite side of the pelvis if necessary. Imagine a position that looks like the number 4. It is different from the posterior impingement test because

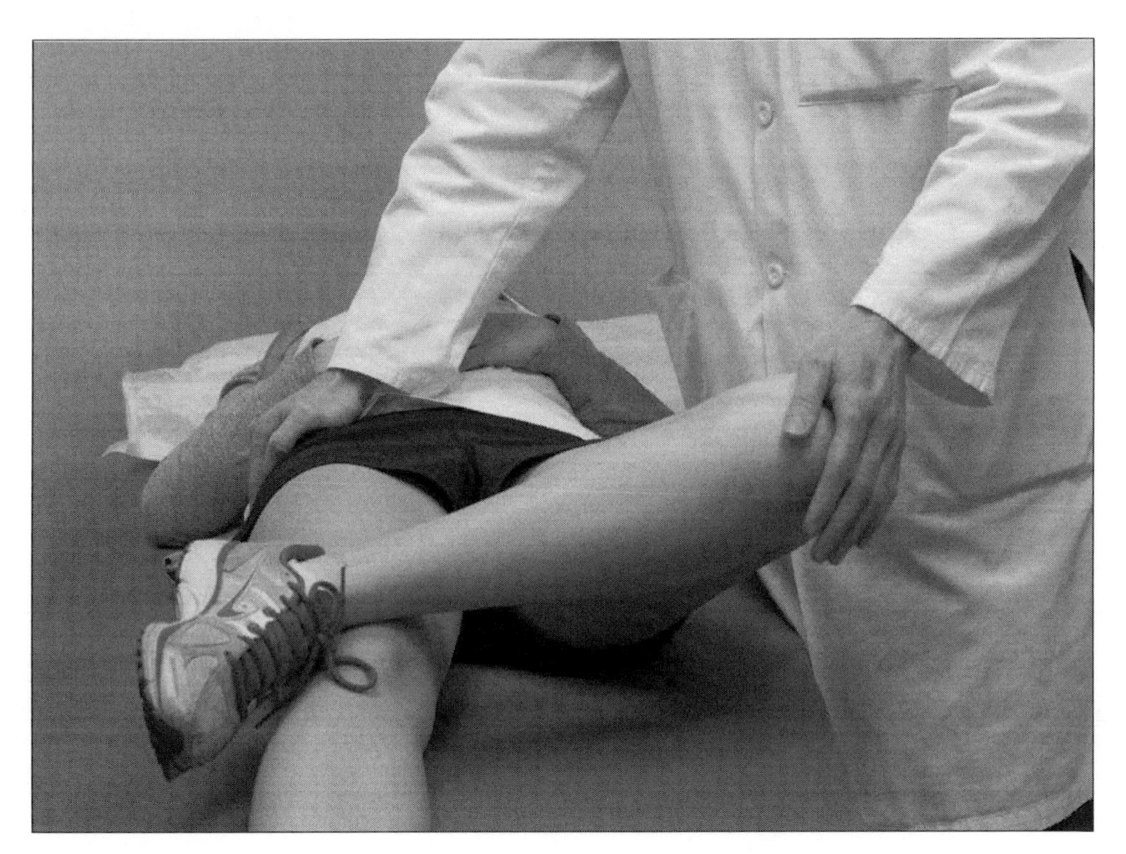

Figure 20: The FABER test
Photography by Jeffery Newburn.

the leg is flexed instead of extended. While the leg is in the figure 4 position, your physician will measure the so-called FABER's distance from the side of the knee to the examination bed (6). *See Figure 20.*

A positive FABER test is defined as any loss of distance between the side of the knee and the table. If there is an unaffected hip the difference between hips can be significant. The 2007 study mentioned earlier found that 97 percent of the patients had a positive FABER test. The significance of the FABER test in terms of actual bony impingement is not clear according to the study results. Whereas it was clear that the FABER test was positive in most of the patients, the hip arthroscopies were not able to correlate the loss of motion measured during the test to a direct mechanical impingement cause. The researchers felt that the loss of motion was mainly due to apprehension. Nevertheless, after the surgeries to correct FAI the FABER's distance improved in the patients participating in the study (the study results did not state in how many patients FABER's distance improved) (3).

Could part of that apprehension be caused by, for example, restricted adductors, hip flexors and buttock pain? Could the root cause have been relieved by the surgery and tightness etc.

addressed in physical therapy? Having been an FAI patient, my own experience says yes. It remains to be seen what future studies say on the significance of the FABER test for FAI.

According to FAI specialist Dr. Chad Hanson, the FABER test fulfills another function, as it may indicate iliopsoas strain or contracture: "In some patients with severe pain inside the hip, their knee may point almost straight up to the ceiling. Patients that have a bad FABER test and have pain when they go from flexion to extension are patients that I will keep in the back of my head that may require further investigation as to the percentage involvement of the psoas" (6).

If the FABER test reproduces groin pain, the test can also help indicate an iliopsoas (hip flexor) strain or a disorder in the hip other than FAI (15).

6.3.1.4 General Testing

At some point during your visit the doctor should also check some general landmarks like your range of motion (ROM), look for generalized instability (lax ligaments), evaluate the lower spine and make sure your neurological signs are intact, and check if your sacroiliac (SI) joints are stable. SI joints are the ligamentous joints connecting each side of the sacrum, below the lumbar spine, to the largest pelvic bone, called the ilium. After the anterior and posterior impingement tests, the FABER and the generalized testing, the physician should have a clear picture of the severity of your pain. It's time to get some imaging.

6.3.2 Imaging

A natural part of getting or making a diagnosis of hip impingement will be to obtain imaging of the hips. There are different kinds of imaging that may be helpful. If you are like me and have not been accurately diagnosed for a long time, you might already have obtained imaging of various parts of your body where you have pain, like sacroiliac joints (pelvis), knee, or even lumbar spine. In many cases, imaging those parts that hurt might produce perfectly normal readings, like "unremarkable sacroiliac joints," maybe some minor "degenerative disc disease" in the lumbar spine or "intact ligaments" of the knee joint. Such normal readings may occur if the true cause of your pain is FAI. I'm not saying that you couldn't have multiple pathologies (diseases); the trick is to determine which ones are producing what pain.

As previously mentioned, a significant number of lumbar spine MRIs show a false-positive, meaning that the MRI reading may say degenerative disc disease. Unless you can clinically correlate the MRI findings to your pain (for example, a nerve block that turns off radiating leg pain or a diagnostic hip joint injection that helps your hip pain), a positive MRI finding, be it in the lumbar spine or the hip joint, probably isn't the source of your pain. I have chosen to include this more general information because of my experience with pain management specialists. Some of them love to shoot you up with injections based on an MRI reading, even when the pain pattern does not correlate to the MRI.

However, now that you have hopefully found an FAI specialist, you should expect to get the right kind of imaging. That said, it is worth mentioning a 2011 study by the Hospital for Specialty Surgery in New York (HSS). The study's objective was to determine which imaging findings correlate with, and are predictive of, hip pain in FAI. One hundred prospective patients with clinical and radiographic findings of one-sided FAI symptoms were included in this study. All of them filled out a pain questionnaire. Two independent-blinded surgeons then assessed antero-posterior (front-back), AP, and lateral (side) radiographs using 33 radiographic parameters of FAI.

The study's authors calculated correlations between pain scores and radiographic findings. A matched radiographic analysis compared painful versus pain-free hips. The study also compared males and females. When compared to the pain-free hip in the same patient, a painful hip was shown to have a lower neck shaft angle, a greater distance from the ilioischial line (where the ilium meets the ischium in the hip joint) to the acetabular fossa (a circular indentation at the deepest point of the hip socket), and a larger distance from the cross-over sign to the superolateral (upper side) point of the hip socket. Symptomatic hips in males had more joint space narrowing, femoral bone spurs, higher α-angles and larger, more ill-fitting femoral heads compared to females. Females had more medial acetabular fossa relative to the ilioischial line and a lower femoral head extrusion index (16).

Similar to other musculoskeletal conditions, radiographic findings of FAI are poor predictors of hip pain... imaging is only one part of making the FAI diagnosis.

That was a lot of medical terminology, and you don't need to understand every word to understand the conclusion of the study: Similar to other musculoskeletal conditions, radiographic findings of FAI are poor predictors of hip pain. One limitation of the study is that you don't know if a pain-free hip will become symptomatic in the future. In other words, you might not have pain today, but will you tomorrow? But, the study goes to prove an important point: imaging is only one part of making the FAI diagnosis. A doctor who is only looking at imaging and willing to treat the MRI may not have the full knowledge of FAI to perform the correct tests to correlate symptoms, much less the specialized skills needed to treat it.

6.3.2.1 X-ray

The most basic imaging is a plain-old x-ray (also called radiograph). It doesn't show soft tissue (cartilage, labrum, muscles, ligaments etc.), but it does show bone and gives the doctor an idea of how much joint space you have and if any arthritis is present. Typically, surgeons require at least two millimeters of joint space to treat FAI surgically. The Tonnis scale is often used to indicate the level of osteoarthritis, if any, in the hip joint. Surgeons commonly say that a Tonnis grade II or III (stages of advanced osteoarthritis) is a contraindication to successfully treat FAI (6). In the section on CAM lesions, I mentioned that CAM impingement lesions are the easiest lesions to find on imaging. Large CAM lesions usually appear on x-rays, but if the CAM lesion is small or is located in the back of the joint, it will not be easy to see on an x-ray. If there is a lot of over coverage on the hip socket (pincer), it may be visible on an x-ray.

Your doctor will probably order an x-ray examination called AP pelvis (anterior posterior pelvis) and also a side (cross-table lateral) view of the hip. Those two views together will allow him or her to take a variety of measurements. Looking at the AP pelvis view the doctor can evaluate you for presence of both pincer (socket overhang) and CAM impingement. If you feel like learning some medical speak, another way of saying CAM is "decreased offset of the femoral head-neck junction." Depending on the view of the pelvis and hip, the doctor can see the offset in different locations of the ball (top, front, side). Whether any of the following are present or not, the AP pelvis x-ray view also gives your doctor the opportunity to look for several anatomical occurrences, like coxa profunda, acetabular protrusion and acetabular retroversion (3).

In a normal hip, the AP pelvis view will show the acetabular fossa line (the fossa is an indentation in the floor of the hip socket) next to the ilioischial line (where ilium and ischium meet in the hip joint). Coxa profunda occurs when the floor of the acetabular fossa overlaps the ilioischial line medially (toward the middle of the body). Acetabular protrusion occurs when the femoral head overlaps the ilioischial line medially (toward the middle of the body).

Any α-angle that is greater than 50° or 55° degrees is considered abnormal and an indication of impingement.

On a side-view x-ray, the doctor can see the α-angle (alpha angle). The α-angle helps quantify the deformity at the junction of the head and neck of the thighbone. Using an MRI to measure the α-angle is most accurate, but an x-ray can also give a good indication. The doctor will draw a line from the center of the head of the thighbone through the center of the neck of the thighbone; then a line from the center of the head of the thighbone to the junction of the head and neck, which is found by the point at which the neck separates from a circle drawn around the head of the thighbone. Any α-angle that is greater than 50° or 55° degrees is considered abnormal and an indication of impingement (5).

There are a variety of measurements your doctor can use to determine if you have hip dysplasia, for example, the center edge angle on the side and front view x-rays. The center edge angle is used to look at the amount of hip socket (acetabular) coverage a person has and rule hip dysplasia in or out. If the angle is low, less than 25°, there is a predisposition for hip dysplasia and hip joint instability. If there are no clear signs of bony impingement or dysplasia on the x-ray, the doctor will probably send you for a course of physical therapy to shore up any deficits or weaknesses in certain muscle groups s/he may have found during the physical exam. If there is no improvement from physical therapy, or if you have already seen several doctors

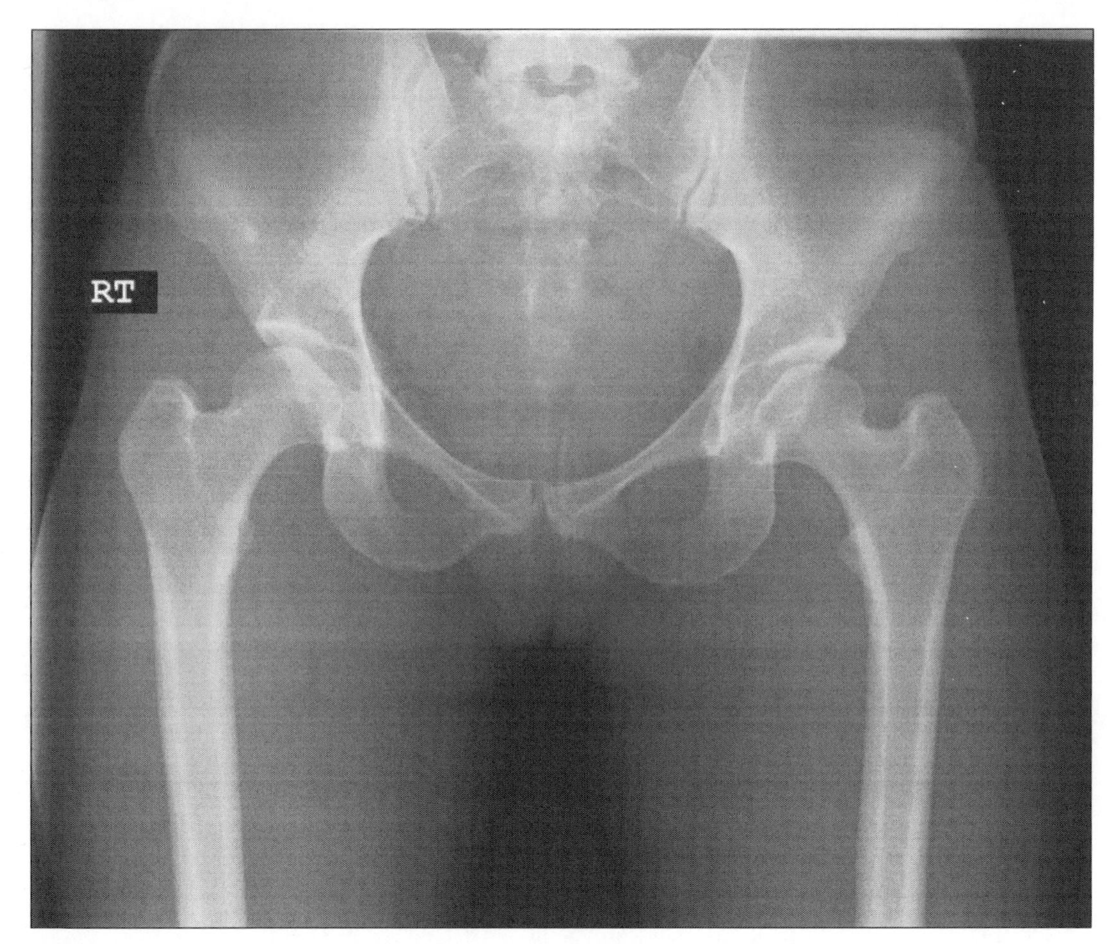

Figure 21: X-ray showing dysplasia in right hip

with this problem, the next step is to get advanced imaging with either a Magnetic Resonance Imaging (MRI) or an MRI arthrogram (6). *See Figure 21.*

Even if your x-ray already shows that you have FAI, the next step would be to perform an MRI scan, so that tears of the labrum in the hip joint(s) can be detected. Some physicians are proponents of computer-assisted tomography (CT) as a technique to visualize the hip joint. The benefits and downsides of those imaging techniques will be reviewed in the following subchapters.

6.3.2.2 *Magnetic Resonance Imaging*

Although CT scans can sometimes be used, most FAI surgeons consider the MRI the gold standard. In addition to bone, MRIs show the soft tissues in and around the hip joint. In order to obtain a sufficient picture of the cartilage and labrum inside the hip joint, there are a couple of options. You can either get an MRI on a strong magnet (3 Tesla or higher) MRI machine, on a lower strength (1 or 1.5 Tesla) magnet machine coupled with an arthrogram — a contrast injection into the hip joint. The 3 Tesla machine has a much stronger magnet and shows a much clearer picture than a 1 Tesla MRI machine. A 3 Tesla magnet MRI machine is not available everywhere.

Some imaging centers have switched to using at least a 3 Tesla magnet. When you use a 3 Tesla magnet, the need for using a contrast dye is eliminated, allowing the radiologist and your physician to look at the cartilage, labrum and signs of FAI in a non-invasive fashion. The concern that some physicians have with an arthrogram is that it is more invasive and involves the introduction of an irritant, through a needle, which can potentially cause pain and discomfort to the patient, without necessarily improving the diagnosis (6).

Keep in mind that MRIs are good but not perfect. Depending on the skills of the MRI tech, MRIs vary in exactness.

If a 3 Tesla is not available in your area, you can go for a weaker magnet MRI; but make sure the arthrogram injection is ordered in addition to the MRI. For the arthrogram, a radiologist will use x-ray fluoroscopy to guide him or her in inserting the needle close to the hip joint to inject a contrast solution (dye) into the joint. The contrast solution helps with visualizing the cartilage and labrum. It will help identify labral tears and cartilage defects such as cysts. It can also help visualize scar tissue that may be present in the hip joint if you have had previous surgery in that joint. Immediately following the injection, you will be taken for the MRI of your hip. Although you will generally not be sedated for this procedure, which in my experience is not necessary unless you are claustrophobic, the imaging clinic will probably require you to get a driver to take you home. After the contrast solution has been injected, you can expect your hip joint to feel thick and full because it is literally full of liquid. It feels like there is swelling on the inside and can remain quite painful for the rest of the day. However, everyone tolerates it differently. Some centers may also require that you stop all anti-inflammatories for several days prior to the injection.

In 2011, the Faculty of Health at the University of East Anglia in Norwich, United Kingdom, performed a meta-analysis (a study to analyze various studies) of radiology studies. Looking at the efficacy of MRI vs. MRI arthrograms in diagnosing conditions in the hip, they analyzed 19 papers, 16 covering MRIs and three covering MRI arthrograms. Among the papers that looked at MRIs only, a variety of machines from 0.5 Tesla all the way to 3 Tesla was used. The Norwich researchers concluded that the MRI arthrogram is slightly superior at diagnosing labral tears in these cases (17). Hip arthroscopist Dr. Chad Hanson says we are still waiting on the literature to support the recent move toward a less invasive diagnostic modality (6).

Keep in mind that MRIs are good but not perfect. Depending on the skills of the MRI tech, MRIs vary in exactness. Sometimes, MRIs lead physicians to underestimate the pathology in and around the hip joint. For example, labral tears or the severity of labral tears are often under-

ted as a result of MRIs. Dr. Chad Hanson explained "you can go into a surgery thinking oing to see a small tear, but you may find a labrum that is completely shredded" (6).

omputer-Assisted Tomography

Some physicians advocate the use of CT scans and 3D reconstructions of the hip joint to better understand the bony components (the impingement). CT does provide excellent 3D pictures of the hip. The downside is that the patient is exposed to a significant amount of radiation. Dr. Chad Hanson said of the use of CT scans: "Our concern for patients getting too much radiation has definitely increased compared to where it was 5 or 10 years ago. In addition, some of the diagnosis is functional during surgery. As you take the hip though a range of motion during arthroscopy you see the labrum getting pinched under and puckered out as the bone pushes up against it. Even with perfect imaging you can see most of the lesions, but not all. I'm warming up to CT. It is an exciting avenue for mapping lesions. The tricky part is tempering that excitement with the realization that you are exposing the patient to a fair amount of radiation, especially if you are getting pre-operative CT scans and post-operative CT scans to measure the amount of resection [bone shaving] that was performed. Is the amount of improvement of the resection enough to justify the radiation? Are we increasing our patients' cancer risk with these CT scans? Or can we improve MRI to the point, with radio sequences or other views, where we can eliminate the need for any radiation?" (6)

6.3.2.4 *Radiologist Competence*

Something I never thought much about, was how competent a radiologist may be at reading films. For the longest time, I somehow assumed that they would all be equally skilled, but why would they? Just like orthopedic surgeons or family physicians, radiologists have different skill levels or interests. As an FAI patient, there are things you should look for in a radiologist. A specialized FAI surgeon should be able to direct you to his preferred imaging center with good radiologists. Unfortunately, insurance companies or geographic challenges can leave us with limited options. Either way, it is a good thing to understand what you should expect from the imaging and the radiologist's report in order to get a diagnosis as accurate as possible.

Preferably, you want to find a radiologist who really understands hip pathology, is up-to-date on the literature on hip pathology and is fellowship-trained in musculoskeletal radiology. With that background the radiologist will have seen a lot of MRIs and know what s/he is looking for. You definitely want more than a two-word report, saying "negative MRI." You want the radiologist to go through the components of the joint being imaged and talk about the osseous structures (bone tissue), provide the α-angle and the center-to-edge angle, look at each of the muscle groups, evaluate the labrum and cartilage, check for scar tissue, and look at the joint capsule.

You should expect a very detailed report from the radiologist since the hip is a deep, complex structure and a challenge to treat. So, if the choice of imaging company and radiologist falls on you, you will want to do your homework. Check which imaging centers are covered by your insurance network, and start making phone calls. The person at the front desk probably won't know the answers you need, so you will have to ask your way to a clinician or manager. Questions to ask could be:

Who of your MRI techs is most familiar with the imaging, sequencing and positioning for femoroacetabular impingement?

Who of your radiologists is a fellowship-trained musculoskeletal radiologist?

Who of your radiologists is specialized in hip pathology in general and hip impingement in particular?

Who of your most suitable radiologists writes the most thorough and detailed reports?

If there is a radiologist who meets my needs, and can I request that radiologist to read and supervise my imaging?

6.3.3 *Diagnostic Pain Injections*

For patients who fail a conservative course of treatment or have a long history of unresolved pain, a diagnostic pain injection can help correlate MRI findings with their symptoms. You should question your chance of success from a hip arthroscopy if you don't have a good response to the pain injection. The pain injection typically consists of a steroid and a numbing medication injected into the hip joint. Even if it is only for a brief period, the injection should relieve a good percentage, if not all, of your pain (6). In the following section, I will provide some ideas on how to receive the greatest diagnostic benefit from a pain injection. Sometimes, the difference in pain is so remarkable, that no tricks are needed, but there may be cases when patients need a little help along the way, to tell if the pain goes away.

Often, the MRI arthogram is combined with an injection of anesthetic (numbing medication) into your hip joint. It is beneficial if the numbing medication mix contains Marcaine,® because the numbing effect lasts longer than just Lidocaine®. From my experience, combining the anesthetic injection with the arthrogram was not helpful. At first, my doctor ordered the MRI arthrogram together with the diagnostic injection. The contrast solution did what it was supposed to do. It completely filled the hip joint with fluid, so the joint felt extremely swollen and brought with it a whole new dimension of pain. It is also possible that the inflamed psoas muscle was irritated by the needle, making the pain worse. In my case, the diagnostic effect of the anesthetic was clouded by needle- and fluid-induced pain. My hip joints hurt so much that I couldn't tell if I had any relief from the diagnostic injection.

My doctor and I decided that we would repeat the diagnostic injections two weeks later, letting the hip joints calm down after the arthrogram injections. We did one hip at a time, and the radiologist used only numbing medication, no steroid. Because my pain was mostly induced by certain movements of the hip, my doctor and I chose to schedule the injections on days when he was available to perform an interval examination (anterior and posterior impingement tests) almost immediately. Following the new round of diagnostic injections, my husband came to pick me up from the imaging center to take me to the doctor's office. He was quite surprised to see a big smile on my face as he pulled up to the curb. I'd been standing out there doing all kinds of gymnastic exercises using my hips, incredibly excited that a lot of the pain was gone.

Once at the doctor's office, my physician performed the same kind of pain tests he had done during my previous visits. There was a striking difference in pain inside the joint — I had just about forgotten what healthy hips could actually feel like. Notably, I still had groin pain at the adductor attachments, but the pain inside the joint was gone, an indication that not all my groin pain was referred from the hip joint. But the pain-free movement of the hip was quite apparent.

Separating the arthrogram and the pain injection worked for me, and begs the question if maybe more patients would benefit from such separation.

Separating the arthrogram and the pain injection worked for me, and begs the question if maybe more patients would benefit from such separation. According to Dr. Hanson, the pain from an injection may vary a great deal depending on the radiologist's technique and where the needle goes in. However, the volume of dye and contrast can be irritating to the hip, the capsule and joint lining. The fluid can offset any diagnostic benefit from the Lidocaine® and/or Marcaine®. In Dr. Hanson's practice it is now standard procedure to separate the arthrogram from the diagnostic injection (6).

Based on my experience, if you and your doctor decide that you are going to get both an MR arthrogram and diagnostic injections done, I recommend doing them at separate occasions so that you are given the best possible opportunity to distinguish pain vs. non-pain. If your pain is always worse with movement, you can try to aggravate the pain yourself before your injection. Or, you can ask your doctor to perform pain tests on you in his office before the numbing medication from the injection wears off. This will give you a fair shot at knowing what really hurts and what doesn't.

While my latest set of diagnostic injections performed at the end of 2010 was really helpful in determining pain coming from the hip joint, I want to share with you an experience from a previous diagnostic injection, performed in 2006, which turned out to be quite useless. In June of 2005, I suffered a still to-this-day undiagnosed soft tissue injury in the groin area, probably secondary to FAI. At the time of the diagnostic hip joint injection in 2006, I still had lots of soft tissue pain from the injury. Needless to say, if the soft tissue pain were not referred from the hip joint, then an injection of anesthetic into the hip joint wouldn't affect that pain. At that time, I was not able to distinguish the soft tissue pain from the movement-induced FAI pain, and I did not know how to look for it. At my follow-up visit, I told the doctor that I still had pain. Based on the information I gave him, he did not pursue the MRI arthrogram. Not knowing any better, I didn't insist.

In retrospect, I'm angry with myself for not insisting on an arthrogram MRI. What did I know? I had never heard of FAI or labral tears. The MRI showed a normal joint. x-rays were normal. The diagnostic injection did not relieve pain, and hip problems were just for older people, right? I now see that it was probably a good thing I didn't get the MRI arthrogram back in 2006. Had it shown a labral tear, the orthopedic doctor may have talked me in to letting him repair it, but he would not have been qualified to treat the bony impingement. As frustrating as it is to know that I did not receive the medical care I needed, I thank my lucky star that no one but my current orthopedic surgeon got the opportunity to operate on my hips.

6.4 Diagnostic Challenges

Being diagnosed with FAI can actually be relatively easy if you 1) find the right doctor, 2) have clearly visible cam or pincer lesions on x-ray or MRI, 3) your pain is very typical of hip pain and 4) you have a clearly decreased range of motion. But hip patients are more complex than that — our symptoms can vary, even if we share an underlying condition. In the following section, I will review some factors that may make it harder to diagnose FAI.

6.4.1 Hypermobility

With hip impingement, joint hypermobility or ligament laxity can be an issue that further complicates diagnosing FAI. As I mentioned under General Testing, your surgeon should include a test for hypermobility when evaluating you for hip impingement. There are different grades of hypermobility, ranging from having slightly lax ligaments to severe disorders of the connective tissue.

Your doctor might use a simple a test called Beighton's Score or 5 Signs of Laxity to determine if you have a level of ligament laxity. The five signs include touching your thumb back to your forearm, hyperextending the pinky finger, hyperextending the elbows, hyperextending the knees, and being able to put your palms on the ground without bending your knees. If these tests are positive, that is an indication of instability (i.e., a score greater than 6 out of 9). If you have three out of five signs, you may be at risk of having laxity, which may make the outcome of a labral repair more uncertain. But that doesn't necessarily mean that you are going to re-tear your labrum after surgery (6).

The most extreme situations of hypermobility are found in conditions like Ehlers-Danlos, Marfan or Down's Syndrome, all of which affect the body's connective tissue. Getting a long-term good outcome from surgery to treat FAI is very challenging in patients with such a connective tissue disorder, because the patients do not have enough high quality collagen in their connective tissue. Unfortunately, that makes re-injury to the labrum, even after repair, a real possibility (6).

Depending on your general ligament laxity, FAI causes a more or less limited range of motion at the hip joint. If you have a lot of ligament laxity, but wouldn't be considered a hypermobile person per all the testing criteria, it still can be difficult to get a diagnosis of FAI, because you still have a good range of motion. The ligamentous laxity allows your joints to move well, despite the bony impingement. To evaluate hip stability, your doctor may use a dial test, where you lie with your back on the table and s/he rotates your leg to see how the front of the hip capsule rebounds, and if there is good tension in the soft tissues in the front of the hip. Using the dial test helps to show if a patient has any signs of snapping, either internal or external, and can help the doctor understand the hypermobility. Ligament laxity is definitely a challenge for an early diagnosis. Even for an experienced FAI surgeon, it may be difficult to diagnose FAI during first or second visits (6).

In hypermobile patients or patients with loose ligaments, the labrum has to work a little harder.

Unfortunately, ligamentously lax patients are at a higher risk of hip problems and joint problems in general. In cadaver studies, certain ligaments were cut to create a condition similar to someone who has lax ligaments or does not have quality joint stability. Such studies have led doctors to conclude that, in hypermobile patients or patients with loose ligaments, the labrum has to work a little harder (6). If you recall from earlier, the labrum is like a gasket in the hip that provides the seal and the suction of the joint to maintain a stable socket, keep joint pressure low, lubricate the joint, and decrease the joint friction.

If a patient who already has instability in the joint undergoes arthroscopy to treat FAI, there are ways to treat the instability during surgery. A procedure called capsular plication, or capsulorrhaphy, shrinks the volume of the socket in the capsule, providing more joint stability (18).

Certainly, far from all hip impingement sufferers are hypermobile, and only a fraction of people have a connective tissue disorder. From personal experience, I know how confusing even a tad of hypermobility or ligamentous laxity can be to an orthopedic surgeon if that doctor is not specifically trained in diagnosing and treating FAI. My hip impingement was overlooked time and time again simply because I had good range of motion, at first glance. Attention gymnasts, dancers and other flexible readers - keep hypermobility and its implications on diagnosing FAI in mind if you are struggling with pain that might be caused by the hip joints.

6.4.2 Secondary Injuries and Differential Diagnoses

I have touched on this subject earlier, but as you go about getting a diagnosis for your pain, it is worth mentioning secondary injuries again, because they can be confusing to physicians confronted with a variety of symptoms. When you have FAI, you are likely to alter the biomechanics of your gait. As the labrum becomes less able to do its job, some muscles work harder than they should and muscle imbalances develop. Often, hip impingement sufferers may develop a limp that will continue to throw off the kinetic chain. These biomechanical alterations caused by FAI can create a lot of the secondary problems. For example, partial tears and tendinitis of the gluteus medius and minimus are frequently found in patients with hip impingement. Adductor pain, hip flexor symptoms and hamstring problems are all very common. During the pre-operative examination, your doctor should palpate those sites to see if the muscle palpation correlates to damage on MRIs and to the pain you feel. Sometimes, the damage isn't visible on MRIs, but pain exists from overuse of muscles anyway.

On the one hand, patients whose underlying cause of problems is FAI may run into diagnostic challenges if they are being seen by a doctor who is unable to properly diagnose FAI. The secondary injuries may be diagnosed and treated but not the underlying problem, sometimes leaving the patient on an uncertain path to recovery. On the other hand, if you do see a specialized FAI surgeon, s/he should always keep differential diagnoses in mind. Differential diagnoses mean other possible diagnoses. For instance, if you do not have a long history of hip pain, but you have pain in the sacroiliac area, it would be reasonable for the doctor to consider a sacroiliac joint injection.

Sacroiliitis often mimics symptoms of labral tears. Dr. Chad Hanson mentions that he has seen patients who got 100 percent pain relief with sacroiliac joint injections. He said that "some people have MRI findings in their hips but are asymptomatic, so you always want to correlate what you see on exam with the MRI and the diagnostic injections. On the contrary, if you have pain in your sacroiliac region, but do not get any pain relief from the anesthetic injections in your sacroiliac joints, we can assume that the source of the pain is not the sacroiliac joints themselves. I see a few patients per week who have more of posterior-based symptoms, who have been told they have a back problem or an SI problem. When it's all said and done, it [the pain] is all from their hips." (6)

6.5 Conservative Treatment

For most patients, a course of conservative treatment is important, and there are a percentage of people who do not require surgery. Depending on the findings and your medical history, a course of conservative treatment may be the right choice. If there are no clear signs of bony impingement on the x-ray, your doctor will probably send you for a course of physical therapy to strengthen weak muscle groups in accordance with the findings of the physical exam (6).

6.5.1 Therapeutic Pain Injection

The diagnostic injection previously discussed can also be a therapeutic injection, and part of a pre-operative conservative approach. Some people might even get to the point where they don't need to have surgery if the inflammation in the hip joint calms down. From a patient standpoint, it is useful to know that sometimes, due to variances in anatomy, patients require a separate psoas (hip flexor) injection to help with inflammation.

The psoas muscle runs right next to the hip socket. In up to 15 percent of all patients, the psoas sheath (the sheath is the connective tissue casing that "wraps" a muscle) is continuous with the hip joint. In those people, the anesthetic from a therapeutic injection into the hip joint will also go into the psoas and help with pain originating from the psoas as well as from the hip joint. However, in 85 percent of patients the psoas sheath is not connected with the hip joint. In patients who have a component of psoas-based pain, the doctor will have to perform a separate psoas injection. The tricky part is that, in cases when there is a lot of bursitis or tendinitis, you have to get an MRI to be able to see if the psoas sheath is connected to the hip joint. When used for diagnostic purposes, injecting the psoas muscle is challenging, because it is hard to isolate the muscle and determine what component of a person's pain comes from the psoas (6).

6.5.2 *Physical Therapy*

A round of conservative treatment is the right thing to do if you don't have a long history of undiagnosed hip pain and no clear-cut imaging showing FAI with correlating symptoms. However, when physical therapy is prescribed to you over and over again, without resolution of pain or maybe with worsening pain, that prescription is wrong.

Hip impingement patients frequently experience more pain with exercise and physical therapy. If your muscles, sacroiliac joints and/or groin hurt more (not regular "I'm out of shape soreness"), even from exercise supervised by a physical therapist, then it's time to find out what the underlying condition is. I don't believe the work-through-the-pain-until-you-get-better motto I was served as my only option prior to finding my FAI surgeon and my FAI diagnosis. While it's true that being a couch potato is bad for you, the more exercise you put your hip joints through when your FAI is untreated, the more damage you can do to the joints.

In essence, if your physician doesn't believe that your pain gets worse with exercise or physical therapy, find a doctor who listens and will find the real cause of your pain. Some physicians just send you to more and more physical therapy. When you still have pain, they say you have tried everything, and send you to a pain management specialist. While it is true that he or she does not know what is wrong with you, that doesn't mean that the pain management doctor is going to figure it out either. Many pain specialists will flat out tell you that their job is to treat pain — not to diagnose it — whether they do it with medications or injections. You owe it to yourself to keep searching for the right doctor.

7 SURGERY TO TREAT FAI

Congratulations if you have gotten this far! It means you received a diagnosis, worked through potential insurance issues and are getting ready to have surgery. For some people, the mere thought of surgery and anesthesia is scary. Sure, surgery is not to be taken lightly. And, surgery to correct hip impingement is major surgery. I am not going to tell you that it was easy, because it wasn't. It was hard, especially, while caring for a young child at the same time. The good news is, when I think back and realize that I did two hip surgeries during 2011, I don't think about how hard it was, but how fast time went by and how well it all went. In the following section, I will provide an overview of the surgery, variances in how surgery is performed and different techniques and components your surgeon may choose to use during surgery to correct FAI. In addition, my goal is to give you some very practical ideas on preparing yourself, your house and your family to deal with the time following the surgery.

7.1 Surgery Options

7.1.1 Arthroscopy

Arthroscopy of the hip joint was first described in the 1970s and then further refined in the late 1980s and early 1990s. The procedure has been used much longer in Europe than in the United States. Recent advances in surgical equipment have allowed orthopedic surgeons to treat conditions that were traditionally either ignored or treated with an open procedure. Hip arthroscopy has been slower to evolve than arthroscopy of other joints like the knee and shoulder, because the hip is much deeper inside the body and therefore less accessible (2).

Because the hip is a ball-and-socket joint, it is necessary to put the joint under traction during arthroscopic surgery, to give the surgeon enough space to fit the surgical instruments (like the arthroscope) inside the joint without causing damage to the cartilage and labrum. The doctor makes two to three small incisions, called portals, approximately ¼ inch to ½ inch long, in the skin and muscle layers close to the hip joint. These portals are used to insert the surgical instruments into the joint. The arthroscope is a long, thin camera that allows your surgeon to view the inside of the joint. Your surgeon may use a flow of saline through the hip joint during the procedure, which allows him or her to see the inside of the hip joint better. Fluoroscopy, a type of x-ray, is also used to ensure that your doctor inserts the instruments and arthroscope properly (2).

The arthroscopic hip procedure is normally done as an outpatient surgery, which means that you can go home the same day as your surgery takes place. Doctors seem to have different preferences regarding what type of anesthesia they use. According to the website for the Hospital for Special Surgery in New York, it seems to be standard procedure to use regional anesthesia for hip arthroscopies: "Normally, the patient is under regional anesthesia. Under regional anesthesia, the patient is numbed only from the waist down and does not require a breathing tube." (2).

As a patient of two hip arthroscopies, I can only say "wow"! My first surgery took four hours, and I had full anesthesia. To clarify, the actual surgery took less than four hours, but the procedure requires substantial setup time after you are asleep — placing the you into a traction table, applying traction and making sure the joint is distracted — and before you wake up — removing you from the traction table, putting on anti-rotation boots, etc. Regardless of the actual surgery time, to be awake for that procedure and aware of the surgeon's every move, would have been a frightful experience for me. Even for my second surgery, which only took two and a half hours, those are two and a half hours for which I would rather be completely asleep. Ultimately, the type of anesthesia used should be a matter of patient preference — not doctor preference. We are fortunate to have a choice of anesthesia. My fear of being awake might be the opposite of someone else's fear of being asleep. Also, some people don't tolerate general anesthesia, naturally making regional anesthesia a great alternative.

Hip arthroscopy, or a "hip scope," is a so-called minimally-invasive procedure. That means arthroscopy is not an open surgery procedure. However, surgery is always invasive. Just because a procedure is called minimally invasive that doesn't mean it is easy to perform or easy to recover from. Still, the recovery is generally quicker and risks of complications are typically less than if a large incision is used to access the hip joint. The traction that the hip joint is placed under during arthroscopic surgery usually contributes to a "pinching" feeling in the hip joint, and it can take months for that to go away. But it typically does go away.

7.1.2 *Open Surgery*

As you might already have guessed, if the arthroscopic technique uses incisions that are ¼ inch to ½ inch long, open incisions to access the hip joint will be considerably larger. Using an open incision also involves cutting through more muscles and risking more damage to nerves. If recovery from the arthroscopic method is generally better and quicker, why would some surgeons prefer and propose to do open surgery, you might ask.

Again, it comes down to the doctor's philosophy. Historically, pediatric orthopedic surgeons familiarized themselves with open hip surgical dislocation to treat SCFEs, hip dysplasia etc. They treated lesions through the dislocation approach, where they cut a piece of the trochanter (part of the thighbone) to be able to expose and see the bone. Patients were on crutches for several months. The large scars can also be quite unsightly (6). Open surgery also involves placement of plates and screws that have to be removed in another procedure later on.

There is another risk with open surgery that may not be commonly mentioned to patients: Adhesions (scar tissue) inside the hip joint. A study published in 2009, performed at the University of Bern in Switzerland, used a scoring system called Merle d'Aubigné to assess outcomes after surgery to treat FAI by means of the open technique and hip dislocation. The study concluded that 75 percent to 80 percent of patients reported good to excellent outcomes after open surgery. It also concluded that there may be several reasons for unsatisfactory outcomes, like joint degeneration with formation of bone spurs inside the joint (osteophytes), insufficient treatment of pincer lesions as well as disease of the femoral head and neck (19).

Adhesions in the hip joint as a consequence from open surgery are mentioned as a recent study finding. Contributing to continued hip pain after surgery, adhesions or scar tissue form like strings between the joint capsule and the shaved area on the neck of the thighbone and may lead to impingement. Instead of bony impingement, or in a worst-case scenario, in addition to bony impingement remaining untreated, there may be soft tissue impingement in the form of scar tissue. Adhesions can be detected by means of an MRI paired with an arthrogram (injection of dye) and treated in a procedure called adhesiolysis using radiofrequency shavers during a hip arthroscopy (19). *See Figure 22.*

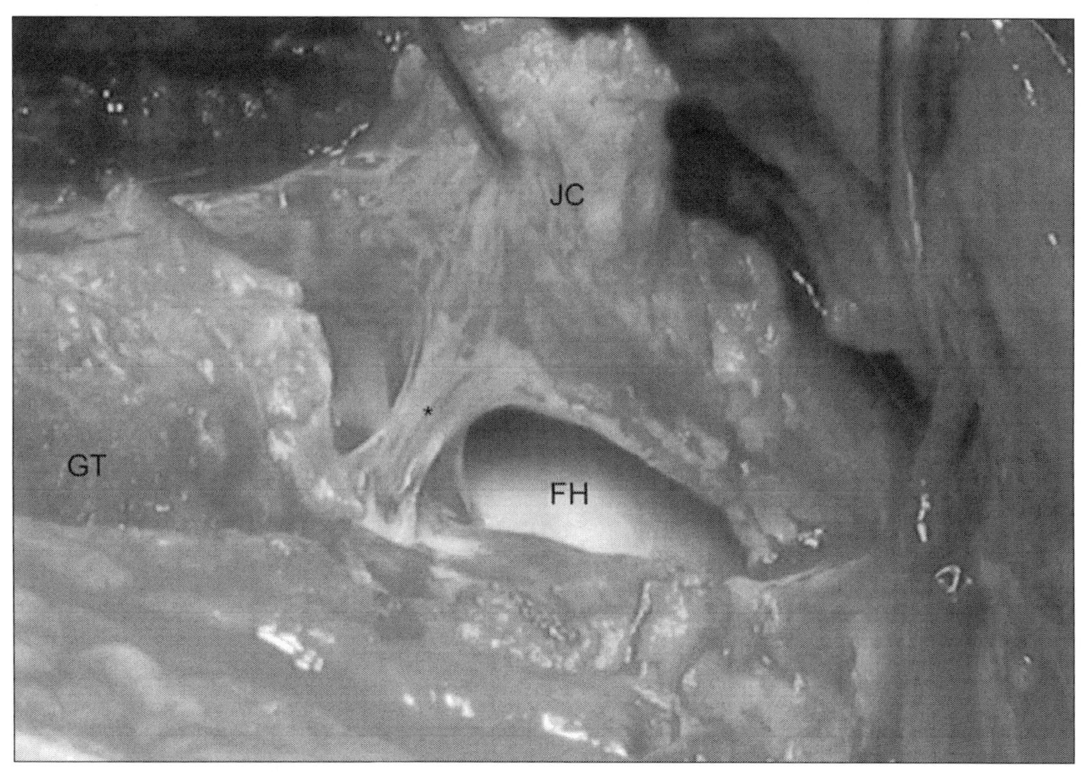

Figure 22: Intraarticular Adhesions Following Open FAI Surgery

Shown is the left hip after open hip surgery to treat FAI. GT: greater trochanter; FH: femoral head (FH); and JC: joint capsule. Adhesions between joint capsule and femoral head neck junction.

Clin Orthop Relat Res. 2009 March; 467(3): 769-774. Martin Beck M.D. Fig. 1. with kind permission from Springer Science+Business Media B.V.

Despite its invasiveness, there is a role for the open surgery, says Dr. Chad Hanson: "I think, for people who have large bony abnormalities, the open surgery is still better able to comprehensively manage the lesion. Arthroscopic surgery is better for more of a limited approach for more of the anterior lesions and less so for the global lesions." (6)

7.2 Surgical Components

During surgery to treat hip impingement, depending on the type of damage you have in the hip joint and your bony structures, your surgeon may perform any of these surgical components: osteoplasty, labral repair and/or debridement, tenotomy of muscle tendons, injections and microfracture.

7.2.1 *Osteoplasty*

Osteoplasty is the medical term for shaving excess bone. Your surgeon will use a number of different shavers, one of which is used to shave away the bump(s) of bone that cause abnormal friction in the joint, leading to labral tears or cartilage damage. In the social media FAI groups that I have followed in the past couple of years, unfortunately I heard about quite a few patients who were left with residual bony impingement after their initial surgery. There is always a risk that your surgeon resects (shaves) too much or not enough bone. As a patient, you are at the mercy of your surgeon. When you select an FAI surgeon, you want to get a clear understanding of his or her osteoplasty (bone resection) approach or technique. Dr. Chad Hanson, who is a Dr. Philippon fellowship graduate, describes his approach to bone resection as follows:

"At the end the end of my cases, I take the hip through the full range of motion and watch the labrum to make sure there are not any further areas of impingement where the labrum is catching or impinged. The mapping [computerized mapping technique] would help to transition this from an art to a science. There has been some work on creating a navigation to help guide the hip resections. However, to be frank, it's not financially lucrative for these companies [makers of surgical equipment] to invest in the technology. Hip replacement surgeons already use navigational equipment because they are putting in a very expensive implant that they [the implant/equipment makers] make money from, so in that area the companies are pushing the navigation equipment. In the area of bone resection of the femoral head neck junction, there is no financial benefit for the companies to push the navigation equipment." (6)

In other words, hip arthroscopy patients will not see new mapping technology in use until there is financial incentive. To me that only proves how important it is to find an FAI surgeon who is highly specialized and trained specifically in FAI and osteoplasty.

7.2.2 *Labral Repair vs. Labral Debridement*

Over the years, treating tears of the labrum has evolved from debridement of the torn portion of the labrum to advanced repair techniques. Numerous studies have compared labral repair and labral debridement. Today, physicians recognize that the labrum plays an important role in stabilizing the hip joint. The consequence of a disrupted labrum may be early degeneration or arthritis. When treating the bony components inside the hip joint, it is therefore crucial to restore the function of the labrum, although the procedure to treat labral tears arthroscopically is a challenge (20).

Patients are sometimes confused about the terminology used around labral repair versus labral debridement. The labrum is continuous with the hip socket (acetabular) cartilage. Your surgeon may choose to do a labral repair with sutures inside the joint or to perform debridement of the labrum. If your surgeon says s/he will do both a repair and a debridement, you might wonder how that is possible. The surgeon is correct in that there is the distinction between labral repair with cartilage debridement and just labral debridement. Let's go over the differences.

Debridement of the labrum (also called resection of the labrum) means that the surgeon resects (shaves) the labrum with arthroscopic shavers.

Labral repair (also called refixation of the labrum) involves repairing the labrum by means of reattaching it with sutures to the hip socket cartilage and bone.

Debridement of cartilage can be performed in addition to repairing the labrum with sutures and involves shaving off some inflamed and frayed joint cartilage, but not the labral cartilage.

So, debridement of cartilage is not the same as debriding the labrum instead of repairing it. From the standpoint of the patient, which one is a more successful approach: Debridement (resection) of the labrum or repair (refixation) of the labrum?

When you select a surgeon to perform FAI surgery, you should ask him/her about his/her philosophy on the labrum and about which technique s/he uses to treat labral tears. Some surgeons believe in repairing all labral tears, whereas some believe in debriding the labrum where it is torn. As a patient you need to consider the function of the labrum when you choose a doctor. Anatomy or technique of this minute level is not often something patients concern themselves with. However, given the variance in outcomes, giving the type of treatment of labral tears a good thought may pay off.

Multiple studies have compared methods and outcomes. A 2006 study of 60 surgeries compared outcomes of labral repair (refixation) and labral debridement (resection) following open surgery to treat FAI. At their one-year follow up the patients in both the debridement and repair groups subjectively described equal improvement. However, at their two-year follow up, there was a clear distinction between the groups. Labral repair patients reported a combined 94 percent incidence of "good and excellent" (80 percent excellent and 14 percent good). Labral debridement patients only reported a combined 76 percent "good and excellent" (28 percent excellent and 48 percent good). Also noteworthy is that the labral repair group did not report any poor outcomes, whereas the labral debridement group had a 4 percent incidence of reported poor outcomes (21).

A later study, published in 2009, compared the outcomes between labral repair and labral debridement during arthroscopic surgery to treat FAI in 75 patients. After one year, both groups showed subjective improvement, but the labral repair group had much better Modified Harris Hip Scores (MHHS) than the labral debridement group (94.3 vs. 88.9). At the two-year follow-up, the difference was even greater; 89.7 percent of the labral repair group reported good to excellent outcomes, compared to 66.7 percent of the labral debridement group (22).

There are quite a few older studies that only examined labral debridement as a technique. Those studies show widely varying subjective results, from very poor outcomes to rather good outcomes. The surgical techniques for both debridement and repair have advanced significantly in the last few years, however, so these studies may not be very good predictors of outcomes from either procedure. Still, a multivariate (looking at more than one statistical variable) study of outcomes following FAI treatment found labral repairs to be an independent predictor of better outcome when compared to labral debridement (20).

Despite the studies that show better outcomes for labral repair, Dr. Chad Hanson emphasizes that you can still get a very good outcome with labral debridement. "There are many who argue that we should do more debridement and fewer repairs. But more of the arthroscopic literature backs that patients tend to do better, in most cases, with the labral repair. When you debride (resect) the labrum you lose the ability to get the suction seal or the gasket effect of that hip. We still don't know the long-term ramifications of performing labrum resections. What we do know, is that labral repairs tend to have a better outcome than debridement of the labrum. Even the longest literature now is not long enough to know if one method is far superior to the other." (6)

There is literature that supports both labral repair and debridement as options for treatments. There are cases where the labrum is simply too damaged to be repaired, where the labrum is so damaged that the torn tissue functions as a loose body. In those cases, the patient would see some benefit to debridement (6).

7.2.3 *Microfracture*

Depending on the amount of degeneration, some FAI patients have already suffered cartilage loss. Research shows that joint cartilage defects seldom heal without a little help. In order to promote the formation of new cartilage where it has been lost, your surgeon might suggest using a technique called microfracture. It is a procedure where your surgeon drills small holes into patches of bare bone inside the hip joint. When successful, microfracture creates a fibro-scar cartilage, which is not as resilient and does not have the same properties as native cartilage. Nevertheless, in the knee, and more recently to a lesser degree in the hip, microfracture has been shown to improve the cartilage coverage.

In theory, microfracture sounds easy, but in reality it is a challenging technique that not every surgeon can perform successfully. The recovery in terms of time on crutches is considerably longer when microfracture is used compared to just osteoplasty and labral repair. Although there are promising studies on microfracture, its efficacy is still uncertain. The Steadman Philippon Research Institute in Colorado performed a micro-study in which nine patients who had undergone hip arthroscopy with microfracture had a second-look arthroscopy of their hips to determine how successful the microfracture had been at reconstructing cartilage. During the primary arthroscopy, the size of the cartilage defect was measured; during the second-look arthroscopy, the percent fill of the defect and repair grade were measured and noted (23).

At the time of the second-look surgery, the average fill of the hip socket cartilage lesions at was 91 percent with a range of 25 percent to 100 percent. One patient only had a 25 percent fill area at second-look as well as osteoarthritis and went on to a total hip replacement. In general, the cartilage defects responded well to microfracture. Eight out of nine patients had 95 percent to 100 percent coverage of an isolated hip socket cartilage lesion or a hip socket lesion associated with a lesion on the femoral head (23).

According to Dr. Chad Hanson, microfracture in the hip is still in its infancy. While it's well understood and can be well executed in the knee, the hip joint is different for many reasons. The thickness of the cartilage in the hip joint is much less than in the knee, and the ability to find a suitable lesion for microfracture is much smaller. "In the knee, we talk about a chondral [joint cartilage] defect, or an area where you are down to bone, as having 'good shoulders,' meaning that there is good cartilage on all sides. With the hip acetabulum [socket], sometimes the cartilage is so thin that you don't really see a well-shouldered lesion that is appropriate for trying to create new cartilage. Microfracture is for focal small defects and not for diffuse cartilage loss. If you have an area smaller than a dime you can consider that for microfracture. Once the area is bigger than that, you are asking a lot of the body, and it could be a challenge to get a good outcome. I seldom use microfracture, only when it is truly indicated." (6)

As a hip impingement patient considering surgery to treat FAI, you will probably want to have a detailed conversation about microfracture with your surgeon if s/he suggests you undergo this procedure. Can s/he see and show you that you have "good shoulders" and that the cartilage defect is not too great to prevent a poor outcome? How often does the surgeon perform microfracture? What have the outcomes been for previous patients? As much as we all want to get better, we also need to make sure that we get the procedures that are the most beneficial to us and don't take us back a step.

7.2.4 Psoas Tenotomy

Tenotomy is the medical term for dividing a muscle tendon. Sometimes the term "release" is used, but the more correct term is probably "fractional lengthening" since only about 50 percent of the muscle tendon sheath is released, or divided, to give more length and flexibility to the muscle. Psoas is a major hip flexor that attaches along the lumbar spine, comes through the pelvis, overlays the hip joint and attaches on the middle of the thigh to a part of the thighbone (the lesser trochanter). If you recall from the paragraphs on FABER Test and Conservative Treatment, the psoas muscle is often involved in and a cause of pain at the hip joint in patients with hip impingement. Given the number of FAI patients who struggle with psoas pain and tightness, I think some of us would even agree to call psoas "a beast."

The FABER test can give your doctor an indication if the psoas causes you pain, but it may be hard for your surgeon to know for sure whether a psoas tenotomy is necessary or not without looking inside the joint. It often takes looking through the arthroscope to see whether there is bruising or tearing on the front of the labrum where the psoas snaps across it. If there are visible signs of psoas impingement, then your surgeon may choose to lengthen this muscle during surgery to correct FAI. In the following section, I will review some of the research presented about psoas tenotomy, who may be a good candidate and different techniques that may be used.

7.2.4.1 Who Is A Candidate for Psoas Tenotomy?

A study presented in 2011 researched who is a good candidate for psoas tenotomy and who is not. In their study, researchers at the Hospital for Special Surgery (HSS) in New York identified a group of patients who may not respond favorably to surgery for a snapping psoas tendon. The study concluded that surgeons should be cautious about releasing the psoas tendon, particularly if there is some structural instability in the hip, and especially if there is decreased femoral anteversion. Although the psoas tendon may be causing pain, it also provides some dynamic support to the hip and may cause problems if it is released (24).

Anteversion means "leaning forward." Femoral anteversion is a condition in which the femoral neck leans forward in relation to the rest of the thighbone. This causes the lower extremity on the affected side to rotate internally (i.e. the knee and foot twist toward the midline of the body). Because some degree of rotation of the thighbone is always present as kids grow, the rotation is considered abnormal only if it is significantly different from the average value of a patient of the same age. Femoral anteversion is very common in children and affects about 10 percent of young children. In 99 percent of these cases the anteversion corrects itself. In any case, femoral anteversion is not necessarily a precursor of future hip problems (25). *See Figure 23.*

The HHS study authors investigated 67 patients who underwent arthroscopic lengthening of a painful psoas tendon. Preoperative CT scans were obtained, and femoral anteversion was used to categorize patients into two groups: 48 patients with low or normal anteversion (<25°) and 19 patients with high anteversion (>25°).

Modified Harris Hip Scores (MHHS) and Hip Outcome Scores (HOS), divided into the subscales Sport and Daily Living, were used to assess preoperative and postoperative outcomes. The study found significant differences between the groups, with the high anteversion group showing a strong association with a worse HOS-Sport subscale — but no difference in the HOS-Activities of Daily Living subscale. On the MHHS questionnaire, the group with high anteversion scored significantly worse with regard to athletic and daily living activities.

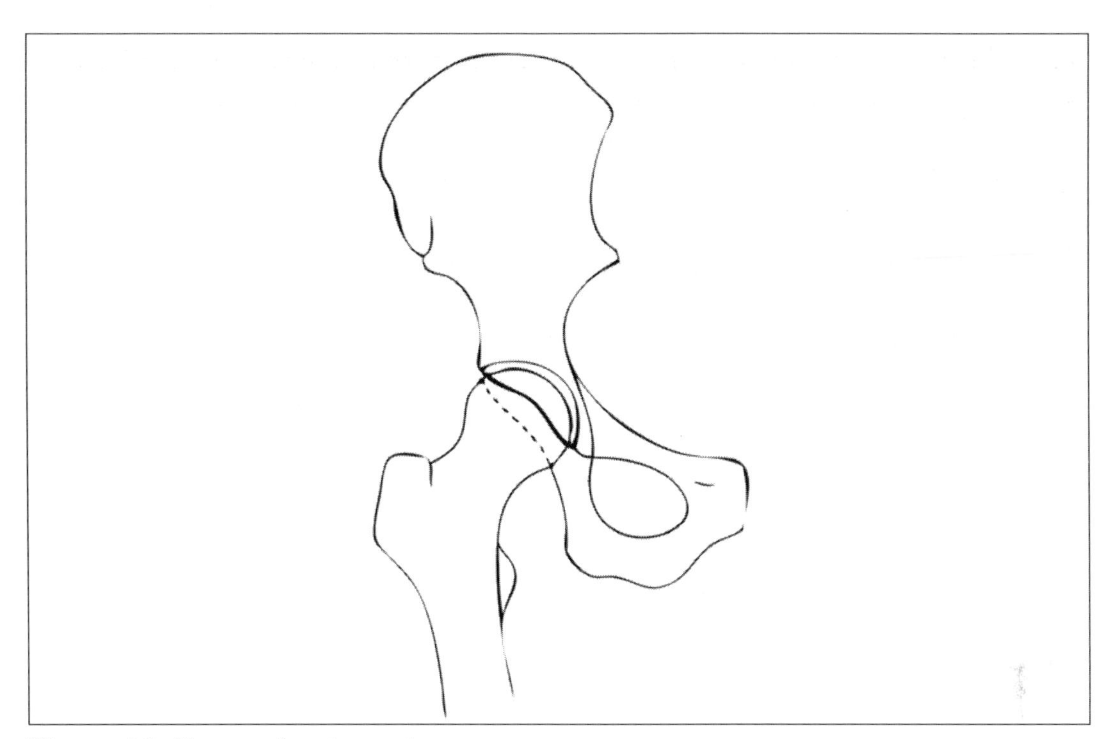

Figure 23: Femoral anteversion

Printed with permission from the *Journal of Bone and Joint Surgery American*, May, 2006, 88, 5, Treatment of femoro-acetabular impingement: preliminary results of labral refixation, Espinosa, 925-935.

In addition, twice as many patients who had high anteversion eventually had to undergo revision surgery (24).

7.2.4.2 Psoas Tenotomy Techniques

Surgeons may use different techniques for releasing the psoas muscle. The question is: does it make a difference at what part of the muscle psoas is released? Dr. Thomas Byrd followed 68 hip patients for a minimum of 12 months and up to 24 months after hip arthroscopy and/or endoscopic surgery to treat a snapping psoas tendon. Two techniques were utilized: releasing the tendon from the lesser trochanter via the iliopsoas bursa (21 hips) or release through one of the hip arthroscopy views (47 hips) (26).

According to the study abstract, the average improvement for each hip was 25 points on the Modified Harris Hip Score with the snapping resolved in 95.6 percent of cases. Forty-eight hips had coexistent joint pathology that was treated with arthroscopy. Three patients developed a bone formation outside of normal bone structures, called heterotopic ossification, which required excision; all of these tenotomies had been performed from the site of the lesser trochanter. Four patients also underwent a repeat arthroscopy because their symptoms were not resolved. Dr. Byrd drew the following conclusion: "We reported 96 percent resolution of the snapping, and that is good, but what that means is that we had three patients who we did the operation on and it did not solve their problems. In my mind, that was not a failure of the technique but it was a failure to make the correct diagnosis. That tells me that there is a lot we still do not understand." (26)

A different study looked at three different common types of psoas tenotomies: release at the level of the labrum, at the femoral neck and from the lesser trochanter. The purpose of the study was to determine how much of the muscle-tendon unit (MTU) is released with each one of the techniques. Using cadavers and comparing circumferential measurements of the MTU taken at the different release sites, the study was able to conclude that none of the psoas tenotomy techniques results in a release of the entire MTU.

What is an FAI patient to make of all of this? As a layperson, I cannot tell what limitations the studies suffered from, and if further, larger studies are needed, but the topic is worth a few reflections. First of all, if 10 percent of children have femoral anteversion and it resolves in 99 percent of children, statistically speaking 0.1 percent of adults would have some degree of femoral anteversion unless it is treated during childhood. Considering that femoral anteversion in childhood is not a precursor of future hip problems, this tells us that, although possible, for an adult with hip impingement and/or a snapping iliopsoas tendon to have femoral anteversion it is not very common. But asking if you have femoral anteversion is certainly in order, if your FAI surgeon contemplates a psoas tenotomy.

In addition, all of the patients who underwent psoas tenotomy and developed abnormal bone growth had the tenotomy performed from the lesser trochanter. It wasn't a large study and more research is probably needed. However, I would be inclined to think that psoas tenotomy performed from the lesser trochanter is not as successful as the release from the hip arthroscopy portal at the labrum despite the fact that the site of the release does not seem to matter as far as preserving enough intact entire muscle-tendon unit goes. As a patient, asking your surgeon what approach he or she uses seems appropriate.

7.2.5 *Labral Reconstruction*

When a patient has very little labrum left as a result of degeneration, a procedure called labral reconstruction using an iliotibial (ITB) or hamstring autograft may be used to recreate the suction seal of the hip joint. The iliotibial tract is a connective tissue band on the side of thigh, from hip to knee, often called IT band. In a study performed between 2005 and 2008, Dr. Marc Philippon performed 95 arthroscopic labral reconstructions with ITB autograft in patients with advanced labral degeneration or deficiency. Forty-seven of the patients met the criteria to be included in a study. Of these, four patients went on to have a total hip replacement and were not included in the follow-up. The labral autograft was taken from the ITB and attached to what was left of the labrum with sutures (27). Other FAI specialists have advocated use of hamstring tendons (those also used in ACL reconstructions of the knee) (6).

The modified Harris Hip Score (MHHS) and patient satisfaction were used to measure outcomes after the labral reconstruction surgery. The mean MHHS improved from 62 before surgery to 85 after surgery. Median patient satisfaction was 8 out of 10. The independent predictor of patient satisfaction with outcome after labral reconstruction was age; the mean age at the time of surgery was 37 years. The study results showed that patients who had labral deficiency or advanced labral degeneration had good outcomes and high patient satisfaction after arthroscopic intervention with acetabular labral reconstruction. Lower satisfaction was associated with joint space narrowing and increased age. In addition, patients who were treated within one year of injury had higher MHHSs than patients who waited longer than 1 year — MHHS 93 versus 81 (27).

7.2.6 *Injections*

Therapeutic injections of steroid into inflamed muscles are sometimes performed during surgery to treat FAI. If a pre-surgery MRI shows a lot of tendinitis in an area, your surgeon may suggest a concurrent injection of steroid, which is a potent anti-inflammatory medication. Another injection therapy sometimes mentioned on social media hip forums and hyped by doctors who provide prolotherapy is Platelet-Rich Plasma (PRP).

PRP involves drawing a patient's own blood and extracting a concentrate of blood platelets. The platelets contain growth factors that help the body heal from injuries. When you are injured, your body's disrupted cells start a whole chain of healing reactions by releasing growth factors (protein) that create inflammation. In turn, the inflammation releases more growth factors. During the next phase of healing, collagen starts forming tissue. The blood platelets from the injected PRP contribute to the healing by supplying growth factors.

PRP is not commonly used in the hip joint, but there are promising study results for tendon rupture injuries. In a consensus paper from 2010, funded by the International Olympic Committee, sport physicians from several countries, including FAI specialist Dr. Philippon, concluded that there is a limited amount of basic science research on the influence of PRP on the inflammation and repair of connective tissue. The physicians went on to say that there is an even greater lack of well-conducted clinical studies on how to use PRP to manage sport injuries. Their recommendation was for clinicians to proceed with caution in the use of PRP for sport injuries and that more work needs to be done to create robust clinical trials (28).

7.3 Possible Surgery Complications

As with all surgeries, there is a risk of complications. For hip arthroscopy, the complication risk is calculated at about 1.5 percent and can be anything from nerve injury from the traction or incision to equipment failure. Fracture of the neck of the thighbone caused by shaving too much bone has been reported but the risk is very low. If the blood vessels in the femoral head neck

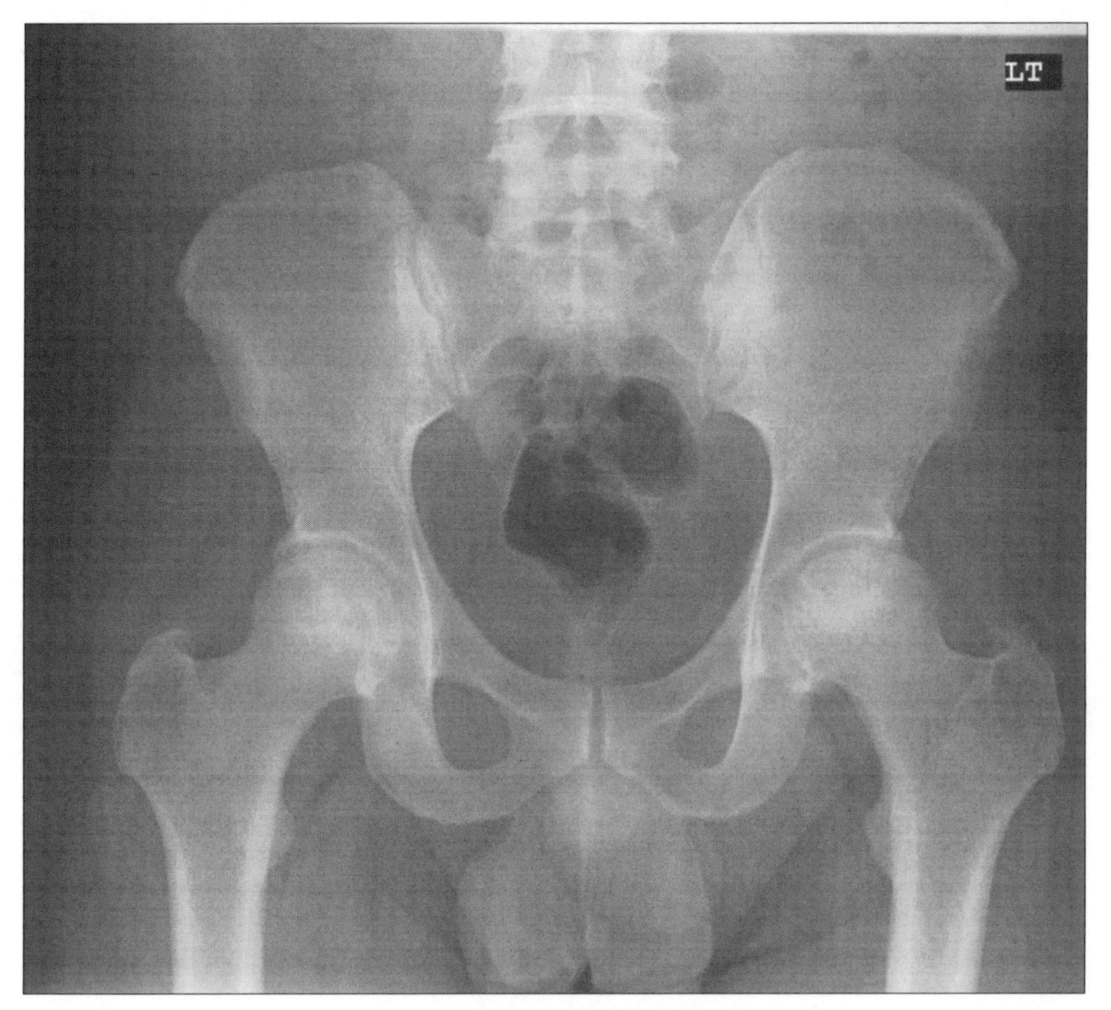

Figure 24: X-ray showing avascular necrosis in left hip

junction become disrupted there is a risk of developing conditions called avascular necrosis or osteonecrosis, which is a lack of blood supply to a part of the hip joint (6). *See Figure 24.*

A more common problem is the formation of adhesions, scar tissue, not so much between the ball and the socket, but in the surrounding tissues next to the labrum and surrounding the joint capsule. Scar tissue can prevent healing and cause pain. You should discuss your surgeon's philosophy on preventing scar tissue from forming with him/her. As mentioned previously, there are different schools of thought on this issue.

Although it may not lead to a serious surgery complication, there is always a risk that the surgeon shaves too much or not enough bone. That in turn could lead to repeated labral tears and require revision surgeries. So if I wasn't clear enough earlier in this chapter, I now want to highlight how important it is that you have a conversation with your FAI surgeon on his method to make sure he doesn't shave too much or too little bone. Unfortunately, inadequate bone resection is one of the most common problems I read about from patients who have already undergone at least one set of arthroscopies, or even open surgery.

Your surgeon should take precautions during surgery to avoid instability of the operated hip joint. The joint capsule plays an important role in providing stability for the hip joint, so finding out what your surgeon's philosophy is on protecting the capsule and the ligaments is essential. You don't want to go from having impingement to having instability, which is considered a surgical complication. Dr. Hanson emphasizes the importance of the capsule: "When the practice of hip arthroscopy started, surgeons were generally happy to get in the joint and repair a labrum and shave some bone. Now we know how important it is to protect the joint capsule and the iliofemoral ligament. We want to minimize trauma to the capsule because the consequence may be that we take a patient from stiffness to gross instability." (6)

7.4 Preparing for Surgery

Getting ready for the first surgery was a big deal. I was nervous. I was stressed out, and did not know what to expect. Oddly enough, I was never very worried about the outcome, but felt quite comfortable with my surgeon's expertise. However, I did worry a lot about my ability to be there for my family, about the post-surgical pain, and about the protective restrictions that I would have to adhere to after surgery.

If anyone had shared with me before my first surgery what I was about to learn, I might have planned some things a little better or differently. For your benefit, I will share my experiences in terms of pain after the surgery, expectations, restrictions and some very practical ideas for making the recovery easier. As trivial as some ideas might seem, some of them were game-changing for my ability to function without more help around the house after my second surgery. Use these ideas as you need them. If nothing else, maybe I can give you a realistic expectation of the recovery phase.

7.4.1 *Get help!*

First, a few words on mental preparation. If you are a neat freak and/or have children, beware! The time after surgery is not the time to worry about cleaning or picking up the house. Make a mental note to accept the mess. It may seem like the whole house is falling apart, but the good news is that about three weeks or so after the surgery, you'll be unbelievably happy that you can clean it.

We were incredibly lucky. My mother flew all the way from Sweden to the United States to come and help us for the first surgery. Afterward, we realized how important her help was for us. By the time the second surgery came around, I was a pro and had learned what steps I should take to make things easier. For that surgery, we were on our own, without any helpful family members, but hired some help. The experiences from the first surgery were invaluable as we were planning out the weeks following surgery number two. Would it have been helpful to have that knowledge even before my first surgery? You bet!

Children add a whole other dimension to your recovery from FAI surgery. Not only do you have to think about who is going to help you after surgery, but also who is going take care of your children. If your spouse or significant other is able take off work for a couple of weeks and adjust his/her work schedule to take over just about 100 percent of what you normally do for/with the kids, then that's great. In reality, that's unlikely to be the case.

In our situation, we already knew my husband's job wouldn't allow him to take off the duration of the recovery. It's incredibly valuable if a family member can come and take over your share. If you don't, when you think about the cost for the surgery and related medical expense, also try to make room in your budget for hiring help.

If you stay at home with little children, you need someone who is going to be able to take over the lifting, changing diapers, and cooking etc. If your little ones go to school, and you are the one who drops them off and picks them up, then you need someone to do that for you. Even when you can drive again, it is scary to take a young child who might run away from you, through a parking lot before you're physically able to run after him or her. Our son went to pre-school during the weekdays, and truthfully it was nice to have peace and quiet in the house — some time for my beat up body to heal and rest.

With the chaotic recovery time from my first surgery fresh in our memories, my husband and I prepared ourselves for the worst. After the first surgery, I had needed a lot of help just for myself for a whole week, which meant that someone else needed to be available for my 2-year old. I was not able to get myself in and out of bed, let alone to get myself into the continuous passive motion (CPM) machine. I needed help to get to the bathroom in the middle of the night, and honestly felt quite helpless.

After my surgeries, I was on crutches for almost three and two weeks respectively. Fortunately for us, the second surgery was easier on me, because there was not as much damage in that hip. I was ready to drop the crutches after two weeks. Less surgical traction time and the absence of a psoas lengthening contributed to the improved recovery time, and I was able to start functioning a lot sooner than after the first surgery. I could even get myself in and out of bed and up in the CPM machine almost the first day after the surgery. That was a huge difference in my need for assistance.

7.4.2 *Helpful tools*

Partly forced by the fact that we didn't have anyone to help us for more than a week after the second surgery, I had to work smarter. Some rather inexpensive and nifty tools helped me perform simple tasks without a helper and made my recovery period easier. With lessons learned from surgery number one, I went on my favorite retail websites and bought a few items of assistance.

Pick-Up Tool

I call it a trash grabber, but it's basically an indispensable tool that helped me pick up all kinds of items from the floor during the hip protective and restricted phase and beyond, when I wasn't able to bend over properly. This tool is also very popular with 2-year old boys who like to use it as a sword and swing it at the plasma TV, so a little caution is recommended. You can, for example, find it online on amazon.com or sometimes in drugstores like Walgreens.

A Good Old Shoehorn

The good old shoehorn is something my dad uses and a great invention. It is hard to get your shoes on before you are allowed to exceed 90-degree flexion at your hip and maybe after that too. With no luxury of a helper at all times, I found a long-stemmed shoehorn to be a reliable companion. Paired with a pair of slip-on, no-tie sneakers, we made a good team.

Raised Toilet Seat and a Shower Chair

At first I felt really old buying a raised toilet seat, but I was really glad I did. It was great for the first couple of weeks, when sitting can be quite painful. I also got myself a sturdy shower chair that was truly an awesome thing to have. I just put it in the shower, jumped in on crutches, sat down and put my crutches away — indispensable.

Wheelchair

For the second surgery, I rented myself a wheelchair. Apart from the fact that the wheelchair previously had been in the possession of a chain smoker and made my painkiller-induced nausea intolerable at times, it made a huge difference in my level of participation in the household. While it's impossible to carry a teacup or a plate when you're on crutches, it's manageable in a wheelchair. An added benefit of a wheelchair is that a mommy-love-hungry 2-year old finds it thrilling to sit on the arm rests. Just make sure you hold on tight.

If your doctor writes you a prescription, insurance companies may cover the wheelchair rental as a durable medical equipment benefit. I ended up paying cash, because not a single in-network business was able to rent me wheelchair. The cost was about $100 for two weeks and that just wasn't the fight to pick. I did end up exchanging the wheelchair for a smoke-free one after a few days. I didn't get the Rolls Royce version, but if you are willing to pay up, you can rent a wheelchair with a tray or a motorized one.

"Euro-Style" Crutches or Forearm Crutches

I am thankful to my surgeon for a lot of knowledge, some apparently more trivial. When I hopped in for my two-week post-operative visit on forearm crutches, he said "oh, you have European crutches." I had no idea they were European, but I guess they really worked for me, not only because I am European, but because the under-arm crutches were killing me. I didn't make it more than two days on the under-arm style crutches they give you at the hospital —

what a horrible invention! They reminded me of a world war military hospital and just gave me incredibly sore armpits.

What types of crutches you use is a matter of preference. If like me, you detest the standard under-arm style they give you at the hospital, know that there is an alternative. Forearm crutches were another out-of-pocket cash expense, though. Be prepared to pad either type of crutch with soft foam, tube socks or other materials that will prevent soreness and blisters. Granted, the forearm style crutches do require you to really use your arm muscles, but that's not a bad thing. These crutches allowed me to move better and more freely, without constant pain under my arms.

Swivel Seat

Another helpful and inexpensive device is a round swivel seat you can put in the car. It helps whether you can drive yourself around or someone has to drive you. When you use crutches to get to the car, you sit down on the swivel seat placed on top of the car seat with your legs hanging over the side of the car. After you put your crutches inside the car and need to move your legs in front of you, the swivel seat helps you rotate yourself without using a whole lot of leg motion. If you have sacroiliac joint pain, the swivel seat can also help you from aggravating the SI pain because you avoid pushing off with your legs, which can throw your sacrum into awkward positions.

Backpack

Whether you hang a little backpack over the handle of a wheelchair or on your back while on crutches, it is of essential value. You won't be able to carry around anything, so a backpack makes life easier for important things like cell phone, wallet and a water bottle.

7.4.3 *Setting up Your Rooms*

I couldn't help it. I had to clean as if I was about to give birth before both surgeries. It turned out that a good non-pregnant pregnancy cleaning was the right thing to do. Once I came back from the hospital, I could actually find the items I needed. Unorganized drawers and closets can be annoying when you are standing on one leg, getting more and more tired as you are looking for something you can't find. A million little toys on the floor are good tripping material for mommy — or daddy — on crutches. Avoid that!

If your doctor orders you a CPM (Continuous Passive Motion) machine you'll be spending a lot of time in your bedroom with your leg in the CPM machine. You might as well set the bedroom up in a way that will maximize your enjoyment of the downtime. I had this idea that I was going to watch a million movies and read at least ten books during convalescence. Well, that didn't quite happen. Life happens whether you just had surgery or not, and your family tends to need you, but I certainly had the luxury of more downtime than I normally do.

Making it easier to get in and out of bed once my hip was restricted, I rearranged our bedsides. For the right leg surgery, I was sleeping on the left side of the bed (the right side if you are standing at the foot of the bed and facing it.). This setup helped to avoid some acrobatics for getting in and out of bed and the CPM machine because I could use my non-operated leg to push off and swing myself around.

Reaching most things you need from your bedside is helpful. I put the bulky cold compression ice machine on a free-standing laptop table that I wheeled to my side of the bed. You might just have to move the whole bed to be able to fit your equipment and yourself with crutches. If you sleep with your leg in the CPM machine, like I did, it will be hard to sleep under a big comforter, so make sure you have multiple blankets you or your helper can rig on top of your leg. The blankets are especially helpful if your foot feels very cold because of poor circulation after surgery.

Three months after the first surgery, I actually reorganized the bedroom all over again to work for the surgery of the left hip. Knowing my help would be more limited this time around, I made sure I had tools like the trash grabber, easily accessible from the bed so I could grab them if I needed to.

Something to consider if you have a low platform bed, is to place bed risers to temporarily raise your bed. If the bed is too low you will be seated too low when you sit down on the bed. Not only will it be extremely hard, if not impossible, during the recovery period, but the flexion at your hip joint will also exceed 90 degrees. Many doctors want you to restrict flexion of your hip to 90 degrees for a several weeks after surgery to protect the joint capsule. Some will even place you in a hip brace that prevents your hip from flexing more than 90 degrees.

Preparing for the second surgery, I even took matters a bit further and put out a week's worth of clothing changes on the surface of a dresser, about waist height. This allowed me to get clothes easily without asking for help, bending to reach drawers or venturing into the walk-in closet on crutches. I pretty much stayed in sweats and t-shirts for a couple of weeks anyway. Looking back, my preparations were well worth the time and cost and made my recovery easier. Of course, you need to decide what's necessary and affordable for you.

7.4.4 Selecting a Physical Therapist

Selecting a physical therapist before you need one is a smart move. Your doctor probably has some suggestions for physical therapists that are well versed with the FAI post-surgical physical therapy protocol, or he or she may just give you a list. Obviously, the more skilled and involved your physical therapist is, the better your chances of coming back quickly and beating muscle imbalances caused by FAI. I highly recommend seeing a physical therapist with experience in surgery to correct FAI and the issues connected with FAI. At the same time, I recommend finding a good therapist who is close to your home. You may be going there quite often, so do not underestimate the convenience of a close therapist. For a while after surgery, it may feel like a major task to get to your physical therapy appointment, so not having to travel far is an advantage.

If you are not sure whom to pick, it may be a good idea to talk to several physical therapists and feel them out: How busy are they? What is their experience with hip arthroscopy patients/FAI and labral tears? Do they perform dry needling and trigger point massage techniques, ART, MAT or similar, which are added benefits? What is their approach to evaluating gait and treating muscle imbalances?

In the process of selecting a physical therapist, keep in mind that physical therapists who rehab total hip replacements, but do not have experience with arthroscopy, may not know what you need. Just because hip arthroscopy is called a minimally invasive technique doesn't mean that the protocol used for hip replacements can be applied to arthroscopy patients. Minimally invasive simply means that it is not open surgery. It is still big surgery, and has its own restrictions and challenges that need to be addressed properly during physical therapy.

> ***Just because hip arthroscopy is called a minimally invasive technique doesn't mean that the physical therapy protocol used for hip replacements can be applied to arthroscopy patients.***

The physical therapist I chose was someone I had known for a couple of years already. I had done both core and hip programs at his practice before my surgeries. In fact, he was the first medical professional ever to mention to me that I may have hip impingement. Choosing this physical therapist made perfect sense to me, because my surgeon also holds him in high regards. In retrospect, although my physical therapist did a great job restoring motion after the surgeries, he is also a very busy therapist. I would say too busy. I would have needed gait evaluation, and more attention paid to treating muscle imbalances. If I were to go back and select a physical therapist again, I would make sure that s/he and I were on the same page of what I expected after the surgery. But no one had written this book for me, and I wasn't really sure what questions to ask or what answers to look for. As usual, make sure your physical therapist is in your insurance plan network or you'll be up for an expensive surprise.

7.4.5 *Take Pre-Surgery Notes!*

A note of advice: write down your symptoms and pain patterns in detail before you have the surgery. As you recover and rehab it is very easy to forget exactly what you experienced before the surgery. By writing it all down, you can look back at your notes and see how you have improved or, let's hope not, have not improved. As I myself am still dealing with some pain, it has been helpful to be able to look back, reflect, compare and make distinctions. If you have to deal with multiple issues and injuries secondary to FAI, writing all your symptoms down before surgery can help to give the surgery a fair shot. This way, you may actually be able to tell to what extent the surgery was a success and what issues, if any, you have to continue working on.

7.5 *What to Expect from Surgery*

Naturally, every surgery is a little different. Every patient is unique, and outcomes may not be identical. There may also be variations in what your doctor asks from you in terms of post-surgical restrictions etc. I was quite nervous and anxious going into my first surgery, because its aftermath was an unknown quantity. Here, I will be sharing some of my experiences, so that you may go into that operating room feeling a little less anxious than I did. My goal is also to shed some light on what patients can expect concerning a long-term outcome.

7.5.1 *Not a Miracle Surgery*

First of all, don't expect immediate results. Some pain may improve right after surgery, but other pain may take a while to go away. Directly referred pain may improve quickly, whereas pain from muscle imbalances may take longer. To use a sports analogy: Hip arthroscopy is not a slam-dunk. Don't expect miracles, but do expect a lot of hard work in physical therapy, good days, bad days, and lots of ups and downs. The good news is, that as times passes, the stiffness from the surgery, the aching and pinching in the joint and, the post-surgical pain become less and less. One day they're gone. That still doesn't mean that you are done rehabbing from the surgery.

Statistics on average improvement can be helpful in setting realistic expectations of your surgery. There are several studies that show an improvement in the range of 25 to 35 points in Modified Harris Hip Scores (MHHS) from pre- to post-operative. If you start before surgery with an MHHS of 45 and end up between 70 and 80 after surgery, that's still not 100 — or a 100.1 if you want to aim for a perfect score — but it is a whole lot better than you were before your surgery (6).

Hip arthroscopy is not a slam-dunk. Don't expect miracles, but do expect a lot of hard work in physical therapy, good days, bad days, and lots of ups and downs.

Originally developed to measure outcomes of hip replacements, the Modified Harris Hip Score isn't a perfect scoring system, especially not for high-functioning athletes. Sometimes the MHHS shows a ceiling effect. Whenever an athlete's function is very high, it is difficult for the MHHS to appreciate how much s/he improved, because his/her function is already much better than that of the main population.

Dr. Chad Hanson said that "objectively, it's difficult to measure progress, but the Modified Harris Hip Score does give a good indication of the improvement you can expect. And, it helps to temper expectations, too. It's important to understand that hip arthroscopy is not a miracle surgery. You are not taking the hip back to a de novo state; you are reconstructing." (6)

Although most patients may have a longer road to recovery, there are sunshine patients, too. Dr. Hanson has seen SI pain (directly referred pain from the hip joint to the sacroiliac joint) resolve as soon as immediately post-op; "I have had patients where most of their pain is posterior. They describe pain when they are in the abducted externally rotated position. In addition, a lot of female patients that have problems with their intimacy will say those problems go away once the surgical pain is gone." (6)

The Modified Harris Hip Score is the most widely used scoring system in studies measuring outcomes of surgery to treat FAI, but it is not the only scoring system. There is also the Hip Outcome Score (HOS), which is typically divided into Sports and Daily Living, and the MAHORN Hip Outcome Tool (MHOT). The Vail Hip Score was developed, and is used, at the Steadman Philippon Research Institute.

7.5.2 *Get in Tune with Your Body*

Unless the surgery leaves you pain-free and without any complaints, you need to get more in tune with your body. If you weren't already, start listening closely to it and pay attention to how certain movements and exercises affect you. In the aftermath of the surgery you will be the most important player in figuring out your muscle imbalances, and communicating with your physical therapist. Depending on your insurance coverage, you may even have to do some exercises yourself once the physical therapy is over. At times, I felt alone, thinking that everyone else must be doing much better than I was. However, my surgeon assured me that there are many patients who still have various pains and muscle imbalances after hip arthroscopy. Most get better and continue to improve for a long time after the surgery. Some patients may have other medical issues or previous injuries that were thought to be caused by the hips, but need to be addressed separately. This is where the pre-surgery list comes in handy, so you can compare all your symptoms from before the surgery with after the surgery. The essence is that you are going to have to continue being your own advocate after the surgery to treat FAI.

However, my surgeon assured me that there are many patients who still have various pains and muscle imbalances after hip arthroscopy.

7.5.3 *Post-Surgical Hip Protective Restrictions*

Different surgeons ask their patients to follow different post-surgical rules and restrictions. My surgeon's protocol follows the Dr. Philippon school of thought, where restrictions after surgery are designed to protect the hip capsule. I will review these restrictions, acknowledging that other patients may be asked to follow a more or less restrictive protocol. In addition, the rules will depend on exactly what procedure is performed. I will go over the restrictions that followed a standard arthroscopy with osteoplasty, labral repair and psoas release.

7.5.3.1 *No External Rotation*

I was required to restrict external rotation of the hip joint for two weeks following arthroscopy. The restriction is in place to minimize stress on your joint capsule, to let it heal properly after your surgeon cuts through it to access the joint. When I was first told that external rotation would be off limits for two weeks, it didn't seem like a big deal. During the surgery, both my feet were placed in anti-rotational boots. The boots were made of a neoprene-like material and separated by a big foam roll to keep my legs properly spaced. Industrial-strength Velcro® straps locked the feet, preventing them from rotating out. Waking up from anesthesia, I soon became aware that I couldn't move my feet. Although my surgeon had told me that this was going to happen, I still hadn't appreciated how uncomfortable it would be.

The boots came off when I left the hospital on crutches, but I was supposed to wear them anytime I laid down to rest or sleep to prevent the hips from going into external rotation. By the time the first night following surgery came around, I no longer thought that avoiding external rotation was no big deal. Try sleeping in one position, without being able to shift your pelvis around even a little bit for two weeks — or even one night! After two days, I called my surgeon who told me that some patients sleep with the operated leg in the CPM machine to prevent the leg from rotating. That was a solution I could (barely) deal with. At least I could move my body a little back and forth and let my non-operated leg fall out to the side or pull it up toward me. When the second surgery came around, I didn't bother with the anti-rotational boots and from the moment I came home from the hospital slept with my leg in the CPM machine.

If you choose to sleep with your leg in the CPM machine, make sure you keep the setting on a slight angle so that your knee is not completely straight — that can hurt, greatly! Or you can do what I did. I kept the CPM machine going for about half the night. That way, I didn't get stiff and could count that toward my total required CPM time. Unless you are completely immune to noise, I recommend earplugs. Sleeping on the operated hip can be tricky during the recovery phase, but if you do, it serves a good purpose. By sleeping on the side of the operated hip, you prevent that side from externally rotating. I actually ended up doing so, especially toward the end of the two weeks of restricted external rotation. If you sleep on the operated hip, make sure your prop yourself up with pillows behind your back so you do not roll onto your back and into external hip rotation.

7.5.3.2 *No Hip Flexion Past 90°*

One of the restrictions your surgeon might ask you to follow is to limit hip flexion to 90 degrees. You might want to think about this rule before your surgery and make sure your house is going to allow you to meet this requirement. Some beds, toilets, sofas etc. are rather low and require you to be seated low. Give your rooms, furniture and equipment some thought when you prepare for the surgery. Think about how you are going to get your shoes and socks on if no one is there to help you. It is better to make appropriate arrangements before you come home from the hospital beat from the surgery. As I mentioned before, some surgeons advocate the usage of a postoperative brace that will actually block you from any flexion beyond 90 degrees.

7.5.3.3 *Restricted Weight-Bearing*

How long doctors choose to restrict weight bearing on the operated hip varies greatly, depending on which procedure is performed. Some surgeons don't require any restricted weight bearing after arthroscopy, while some patients are on crutches for many weeks. The scientific evidence is still not firm, and there are a hundred different protocols for the post-operative period. My surgeon's personal philosophy was to take pressure off the hip while I had the early post-operative swelling and pain, so that I was able to restore range of motion without aggravating my symptoms.

The most common time frame to limit weight bearing ranges from two to three weeks. After two weeks many can start weaning off crutches. Anytime a microfracture is performed, your time on crutches will increase. If your doctor shaves a significant amount of bone (a large bone lesion) you are also likely to stay on crutches for longer, to reduce the stress on the femoral head. Yet again, it comes down to each surgeon's philosophy and preference.

7.6 Recovery

How long you need to recover from FAI surgery is, of course, individual, and much depends on the type of procedure that is performed. Generally, open surgery will result in a longer recovery time than arthroscopic surgery. But that doesn't mean that arthroscopy is easy. The amount of damage in your hip and the techniques used during surgery will all affect your recovery time. After my first arthroscopy, the first week was quite rough, with the second week being noticeably better, but still not easy. Three weeks after surgery, I was off the crutches and feeling tremendously better. After the second arthroscopy, I was already doing quite well just days after surgery. It's important to prepare yourself and your family to allow for sufficient downtime. If your recovery turns out much better than you anticipated, you'll then be pleasantly surprised.

7.6.1 Post-surgical pain

Providing you with a good idea what to expect in terms of post-surgical pain is difficult, since there are probably as many pain levels as patients. So many factors come into play: What type of aches and pains you have going into the surgery, what kind of damage is in your hip, what repairs are performed, your personal pain tolerance, and how you respond to traction. I had a great deal of post-surgical pain from the first surgery, but not very much at all from the second.

I know I'm not the only one who doesn't tolerate narcotic pain medications, and, while I try to get off them as quickly as possible, I don't put pride in avoiding them. My philosophy is that if you need pain relief, it is available; use it so you don't have to suffer. Although I can't say I have ever felt inclined to take more pain medicine than necessary, narcotic medications are habit forming and addictive. Fortunately for me, they make me so nauseated and constipated that staying on them would be foolish. No one really likes to talk about the fact that narcotic pain medicines make most people constipated. So if you didn't already know, and you have never taken any before, be aware that it can happen. For each successive surgery I had done in 2011 — a total of three, because I snuck in a shoulder surgery too — I learned a little better how to prevent constipation. As soon as I came home from the hospital, I began drinking a mix of water and prune juice. It helps, but nothing helps as much as getting off the narcotics.

One type of post-surgical pain that doctors generally do not mention, and that I had not anticipated, was rather impactful sacroiliac (SI) pain and adductor pain. I was nearly freaked out by this new pain. What if something had gotten worse due to the surgery? A week after surgery, I wasn't taking pain pills for hip pain anymore, but to relieve the achiness in the sacroiliac area. Ice felt really good too. A bit freaked out now, I went on various social media hip groups and found that what I was experiencing was actually quite common among arthroscopy patients. Everyone I talked to in our virtual communities said that the SI pain that had been aggravated by the surgery would dissipate after a while. Luckily, it did, after about two weeks. The most likely cause of the pain in the SI area is the traction during surgery. Since I can't prove this, your theory is as good as mine. However, my surgeon agreed that the traction could cause some post-surgical symptoms in the buttocks.

Another unanticipated pain was the burning sensation in the adductor longus tendon at the pubic attachment, which radiated down the inside of the thigh. While that burning pain stayed for several weeks after surgery, it was worst during a few days following surgery. After the most acute pain went away, adductor tightness persisted. The tightness was worse than before the surgery, with sharp pain in the tendon when the legs were butterflied. That pain remained, and needed to be addressed in physical therapy. My goal is certainly not to scare you away from going through with necessary hip surgery, but merely to offer you mental preparation. If your hip symptoms improve, that's worth some post-surgical pain.

7.6.2 How to Care for Young Children during Recovery

I have touched on this subject earlier in this book, but feel it is worth some more consideration as you prepare yourself for surgery. Caring for toddlers when you need someone to help you seems all but impossible. It was definitely hard, although we were lucky to have help. Help is great, but taking care of a young child involves more than just practical, everyday tasks. There is also an emotional aspect to being unable to take care of your child, even if only for a short time.

Young children tend to become attached to the people who help them the most. I got sad when my son stopped asking me for things. He stopped hoping that I was going to lift him up or come get him in the middle of the night. He became grandma's and daddy's boy for quite a while. He would repeatedly call for daddy and reject me well after I was capable of taking care of him again. It took me big chunks of time spent with him for him to stop favoring daddy and let me back in.

Being well prepared for the second surgery improved the recovery, including my experiences with my son. Prior to that surgery, I still worried about not being there for him, but I shouldn't have. Children are very good — much better than adults — at adapting to new situations. Several things helped me bond with my son during recovery: The wheelchair allowed me to help him in ways I would otherwise not have been able to. Knowing that he could come to me and I could pick him up and put him on my lap was a victory.

A dear friend of mine had a great idea, too. Before the surgery, she sent us a gift. It was a new board game with shapes (Colorama by Ravensburg) that could be played in bed, or if I was up for it, at a table. It was great, because 1) it was new and 2) it didn't require me to do anything, but to point and talk. Yet, I was getting involved and able to play with our son. We had something new and fun to do together. After both surgeries, I was able to let our son lie next to me in bed and read a book, and he would fall asleep next to me. If you find the activities or routines that will allow you to give your child some quality attention even during the recovery phase you may feel better about being a mom or a dad.

It is hard when you need to rest, ice or sleep and a two-year old comes jumping at you, and wants your attention, badly. Of course, the other family members are going to drag him or her away to protect you. That's tricky, because you know you can't fix the situation right then, and you feel like you're somehow rejecting your child — at least I did. Keep reminding yourself that your son or daughter will be fine, and so will you. With children, you have to keep the greater goal in mind. After your surgery, when you feel better, you have a greater chance of being a more fun, active and playful mom or dad. You're in it for the long haul with kids, so just do the best you can today.

8 REHABILITATION

Now that you have had the surgery to treat hip impingement, and you are past the recovery phase, your rehabilitation begins. You may start physical therapy as soon as the day after surgery, but the first weeks may be limited to manual circumduction of the hip, isometric exercises and biking without resistance. There is no one chapter on rehabilitation that is going to apply to all patients. Not only do different surgeons have different approaches to rehabilitation, but as patients we also have different problems.

The most common way of defining rehabilitation is as a limited time of physical therapy. Sometimes that is the case. With FAI coming back might often take longer than a simple course of post-surgical physical therapy. Rehabilitation can involve so much more, from self-afflicted exercise programs to dry needling and muscle activation techniques. In the following subchapters I will review the possible components of rehabilitation, and what the entrepreneurial patient can do to improve the outcome of the surgery by staying involved.

8.1 Physical therapy

There are probably as many physical therapy programs out there as FAI surgeons. Just as surgeons have differing opinions on surgery, they also have different approaches to physical therapy. My surgeon definitely belongs to the school of thought that suggests that the sooner you move the joint around after surgery, though with protective restrictions in place, the better. You shouldn't let it get stiff and give scar tissue a chance to develop. When you move the hip joint around, like biking and circumduction do, the joint produces synovial fluid that lubricates the joint.

After both of my hip arthroscopies, I was in physical therapy the day following surgery. I biked on an upright bike for 20 minutes without resistance, with the seat in a position that did not allow the hip to flex past 90 degrees. While I was on crutches the first couple of weeks, I also did isometric strengthening while seated. The sessions would end with the physical therapist performing manual circumduction and internal rotation of the hip, also taking care not to exceed the movement restrictions ordered by my surgeon. I did three months, or close to 40 visits, of physical therapy after each surgery. That may seem like a lot, but was not quite enough to restore full movement in all positions, but with time, I have been able to sit cross-legged and squat on the floor, and all the pinching in the hip joints is gone.

Contrary to my surgeon's approach, some surgeons limit any kind of physical therapy until somewhere around six weeks after the surgery — a completely different philosophy. It is not my job to say who is right or who is wrong, and, as far as I know, patients from both camps have good outcomes. For me, it would have been the wrong thing to not move that hip joint around for so long after the surgery. It only took a weekend of no physical therapy for my hip joint and adductors to feel very stiff. When Monday came, I knew it was time to get to physical therapy, not because my calendar said so, but because my hip was telling me.

The more skilled and involved your physical therapist is, the better your chances of coming back quickly and beating your muscle imbalances are. Yet again, it's important to make a good choice of health care provider. The hip is a complicated structure and requires a lot of attention. If somewhere along the road you feel like your physical therapist isn't working for you, you have no obligation to stick with that therapist. Your physical therapist should follow the post-surgical protocol that your doctor has prescribed and respect the restrictions. Despite the existence of a prescribed program, as an entrepreneurial patient you still have to be involved. Being involved doesn't only mean showing up for your therapy appointments and doing as you are told, but also paying attention to your body and speaking up when something doesn't feel right.

It is important that you let your therapist know how certain exercises affect you. If you keep silent, no one will know how you feel. There may be exercises and stretches that simply hurt in a bad way. Most of the time, your physical therapist can modify your exercises, and sometimes you may just have to skip an exercise or wait until you have recovered more. Starting week three of physical therapy, I was asked to stretch the IT band by crossing one leg in front of the other while standing. No matter how hard I tried, I could not do that stretch effectively until way after my physical therapy ended. The adductor longus tendon simply hurt too much after the surgery. Sometimes, healing just needs time, maybe more time than the number of physical therapy visits your insurance plan covers.

Water therapy can be beneficial when rehabbing from hip surgery. In the water, less stress is put on the joints. You will have to wait until it is safe for you to get in a pool, both from a wound and weight bearing standpoint. Once you are in the water, is important to understand that water therapy is not the same thing as swimming. Just as on dry land you would follow the physical therapy program prescribed by your doctor, water therapy will be subject to a prescription and some restrictions. For example, the breaststroke is something you should avoid for quite a while after hip surgery, since it recruits the adductor muscles to a great extent, and involves excessive external rotation motion. If you have hip flexor tendinitis, the backstroke is a better choice than freestyle kicks. Freestyle kicks engage the hip flexors more than backstroke kicks (6).

Physical therapy is currently an area where there is a lack of unified direction for FAI patients, but it is also one of the aspects of the treatment of FAI that is being researched. The Steadman Philippon Research Institute has undertaken several rehabilitation studies to determine the optimal set of physical therapy exercises for FAI surgery patients. The study results will be reviewed in the following chapter covering muscle imbalances.

8.1.1 *Dry Needling*

Some physical therapists — and some doctors, too — have gone through additional training in dry needling to help their patients heal from soft tissue pain. Far from all physical therapy patients are able to try dry needling, because it may not be available to them, but whether you have had FAI or not, dry needling can be effective in treating soft tissue pain and trigger points. Trigger points are localized tender and painful muscle areas that sometimes feel like knots that, when stimulated, may cause pain elsewhere in the body. When performing dry needling, the physical therapist uses very thin needles much like the ones used for acupuncture (filament needles) to pierce the soft tissues. You might ask yourself how dry needling is different from acupuncture. Depending on whom you ask, the answer will vary. Both techniques employ needles, but acupuncture is based on the principles of Eastern medicine or traditional Chinese Medicine, whereas dry needling is derived from Western principles of anatomy and neurophysiology.

There are two similar but different methods of dry needling. Which method your physical therapist uses depends on where s/he trained. Two schools in Colorado, each teaching a different method, are especially well-known. One method is called Trigger Point Dry Needling and focuses on local pain symptoms in small areas of trigger points, although it may cover many areas. The other method is named Integrative Systemic Dry Needling, which treats both regional symptoms and their pathological influence on the entire musculoskeletal system (29).

I have received both types of dry needling, and the treatments are somewhat different experiences for the patient. For me, both dry needling methods were quite effective in relieving pain. The trigger point dry needling made the muscles jump, more or less, depending on how bad your trigger points and adhesions are in that local area. It's a fascinating sensation, but leaves you quite sore. It's somewhat painful but almost like a good pain. During trigger point dry needling, the physical therapist finds the worst and most painful spots and puts needles in them to make the muscle(s) twitch. The more twitching, the more effective the treatment is the theory.

The integrative systemic approach, which resembles acupuncture, but is still based on Western medicine, is much gentler with hardly any soreness after the treatment. During the needling, the therapist leaves the needles in for a while and there is only occasional muscle twitching. In some areas, the therapist may attach electric current to the needle, to stimulate the nerve that supplies a muscle to get the muscle firing again.

The needling causes an immune response in the body to help it heal. Usually after either type of treatment, I got tired and needed to rest a bit. If dry needling is available where you live, I highly recommend trying it. I had my best post-operative physical therapy weeks when I was able to alternate gentle physical therapy with dry needling sessions.

Effective 2012, the American Physical Therapy Association (APTA) has incorporated dry needling as part of a physical therapist's scope of practice in its handbook. In many states, dry needling is already standard fare on the physical therapist menu, while others still haven't changed their regulations to allow dry needling. Some states are in a legislative grey zone concerning dry needling as part of physical therapy practice, yet others do not have any regulations at all.

If you would like to know if your state allows physical therapists to perform dry needling, you can call your local physical therapy licensing board. If dry needling is allowed, but you haven't encountered a certified physical therapist, the local chapter of APTA might be able help you find one. If your state does not allow dry needling for physical therapists, you might be able to find a doctor who performs dry needling.

In my humble opinion, there is no good reason to disallow physical therapists from performing dry needling. After all, physical therapists perform a lot of other modalities to help with muscle pain. Dry needling just fits in with what they do. In some states there is a political battle with the interests of the acupuncture associations. Could allowing physical therapists to perform dry needling take away some of the acupuncture doctors' business? I really don't think so. Having received both acupuncture and dry needling, they are clearly different schools of thought and application. In addition, physical therapists typically include dry needling as part of a wider treatment or rehabilitation, but not acupuncture.

8.2 Muscle Imbalances

Many FAI patients struggle with muscle imbalances and soft tissue pain. Some seem to get well soon after surgery and complain of little or no muscle pain, while others continue to battle their muscle pain for a long time. If you have suffered from undiagnosed or untreated FAI for a long time, you might have more muscle imbalances than a patient who has had FAI for a shorter time and received an early diagnosis.

Muscle imbalances are an unfortunate consequence of the labrum not working correctly, or of other hip pathologies. In many cases, FAI patients more or less consciously alter their gait, overusing some muscles and underusing others. As a result, some muscles become overly strong or weak and some can develop tendinitis. Your physical therapist is important in helping you address muscle imbalances. However, knowing you may not be able to stay in physical therapy for as long as it takes to correct all muscle imbalances, it becomes your job as the entrepreneurial patient to keep working on — and sometimes figuring out — your specific problem areas.

Although every person is unique, there are some common muscle imbalance patterns associated with FAI. A common pattern for hip patients is weakness or inhibition of the gluteus medius muscle, the strongest hip abductor muscle, accompanied by tendinitis of the iliopsoas muscle. In an article about a study performed at the Steadman Philippon Research Institute, the authors suggest that abductor muscle weakness is functionally linked to iliopsoas tendinitis. The study was performed as a laboratory study using electromyography to determine what exercises are most appropriate for strengthening gluteus medius without aggravating tendinitis of the iliopsoas during the course of a rehabilitation program (30).

The rehabilitation study looked at to what extent each measured exercise activated the gluteus medius muscle and to what extent the same exercise activated the iliopsoas muscle. Based on the results, a set of exercises was recommended for the three different phases of rehabilitation. The phases and recommended exercises are described as follows:

Phase 1: Phase 1 takes place from week one through week four after surgery and up to 8 weeks for a concurrent microfracture procedure. The goals are to ensure mobility of the hip joint and to minimize general muscle atrophy while protecting the repaired joint. In addition, the goal is to reactivate the gluteus medius muscle and avoid external hip rotation past 45° (to protect capsular repair or plication). During phase 1, exercises to help muscle activity initially include isometrics, resisted knee extensions and resisted knee flexion, which activate the gluteus medius slightly. Exercise progression can include double-leg bridges (despite involving hip extension) because this exercise offers controlled motion, moderate activation of gluteus medius and low iliopsoas activation (30). For patients following a Dr. Philippon-inspired rehabilitation program, exercises that require hip extension, external rotation and full weight bearing are avoided during phase 1.

Phase 2: Phase 2 starts week five or week nine (following microfracture) after surgery. The focus is on muscular stabilization of the hip under controlled conditions. The goal is to add hip rotation exercises (short external rotators) and to further develop gluteus medius muscle strengthening. Patients are now fully weight-bearing so that stool hip rotations can be added, where one knee is on a rotating stool and the other leg is on the floor (strengthening the short rotator muscles). To increase the strengthening of gluteus medius hip clams with neutral or flexed hips as well as resisted hip extensions are now allowed, but the study advises to use clam exercises and hip extensions with caution if the patient has iliopsoas tendinitis. In those cases, gluteus medius activation can be increased by side-lying hip abduction exercises sliding the foot against the wall. The foot sliding decreases the force on the iliopsoas (30).

Phase 3: The purpose of exercises during phase 3 is to fully regain strength in the hip joint musculature and to work on strength in both lower extremities. The goals of this phase are to get the gluteus medius back to full strength, and to normalize the co-contraction of the hip abductors and hip adductors to minimize muscle imbalance and get the patient back to playing sports and/or returning to work. During phase 3, prone (lying on stomach) heel squeezes, side-lying hip abduction with internal rotation and single-leg bridges can be started to get a high level of gluteus medius activation and a low level of iliopsoas activation. In addition, closed chain exercises like variations of squatting, leg presses and lunges are initiated to strengthen all of the hips and legs (30).

> Closed chain means that at least one foot is fixed and in contact with the ground or on a machine base, for example, a standing leg press. The foot that is fixed, performs a closed chain exercise. The word chain implies a linkage between two parts of the body like foot and ankle or knee and hip.

Discussing the results of the study, the authors mention hip abduction, either standing, side-lying or with other variations, as one of the most common exercises for strengthening the gluteus medius muscle. The gluteus medius muscle activation was high in the following exercises: side-lying hip abduction with internal rotation, external rotation or sliding the foot along a wall. However, the iliopsoas is much more activated during hip abduction with external rotation. The authors recommend that this exercise be avoided when iliopsoas tendinitis is present. Exercises that include hip flexion or external rotation activate the iliopsoas more than other exercises. While these exercises are unlikely to cause hip flexor tendinitis after surgery, they are likely to aggravate tendinitis that was present before the surgery (30).

Adductor pain is a common complaint among FAI patients. Getting the gluteus medius strong and firing is an important aspect of avoiding overuse of the adductors and getting rid of pain.

In a different study, Dr. Philippon performed a computer simulation to see whether sliding the heel against a wall during a standing leg abduction exercise would reduce force in the iliopsoas muscle and not increase load in the repaired hip joint. Comparing leg abduction alone and leg abduction with the heel in light contact with a wall, muscle and joint loads were calculated. The simulations revealed that sliding the heel against the wall caused the iliopsoas muscle force to drop to a level found during relaxed standing. The wall sliding actually generated higher gluteus medius forces, helping to strengthen that muscle even more. In addition, the heel sliding leg abduction exercise kept the joint load at the same level as standing (31).

In addition to hip flexor tendinitis and gluteus medius weakness, other common muscle imbalance patterns exist. Because the gluteus medius is often weak, there may be a discrepancy between how hard the adductors work and the gluteus medius works compared to what the co-contractions between abductors and adductors should be. Adductor pain is a common complaint among FAI patients. Getting the gluteus medius strong and firing is an important aspect of avoiding overuse of the adductors and getting rid of pain. Another fairly common complaint is that the hamstrings are excessively tight and overworked, while the quadriceps muscles are weak, sometimes resulting in trigger points in the hamstrings and knee pain.

Your physical therapist should be able to identify your muscle imbalances, but ultimately you know your body. You have to pay attention to how you walk and how you use your muscles.

For some patients, correcting muscle imbalances might be more frustrating than recovering from surgery, and is sometimes a process of trial and error. In addition, muscle imbalances are not just about strength, but also about the movement chain and the firing order of muscles. Sometimes muscles have to be retrained to fire in the correct order. Gait analysis is a crucial component in examining in what order muscles fire.

8.2.1 Gait Analysis

I had never thought about how I walk, and no one ever talked to me about it — not even one of all those physical therapists I saw over the years prior to my hip arthroscopies. Not until a friend, who is also an outstanding therapeutic massage therapist, told me what my gait looked like. She has known me almost since the beginning of this whole health care ordeal, and, if anyone does, she has insight into my pain patterns. Once I stopped going to physical therapy after my second hip surgery, I started seeing my friend for massage almost weekly. In a friendly way, she pointed out to me that I walk like a duck.

At first, I didn't get what my friend meant. To me I was walking normally. She demonstrated to me how I was swinging my whole buttock, hip and leg all in one piece. Having never thought much about my gait or stride, I had a hard time understanding how I was supposed to do it any differently. Many FAI patients develop a limp or a gait pattern that helps compensate for the problems inside the hip joint. Even if you undergo the surgeries to treat FAI and do physical therapy afterward, you may have settled into inappropriate patterns of movement that you have to work to break.

Make sure you work with health care professionals who are willing and able to help you with gait analysis and gait correction; it is an important part of rehabilitation. After someone — hopefully your physical therapist — helps you evaluate your gait pattern, you can address your gait deficiencies. I asked my friend how I was supposed to walk. Her answer was "swing both hips - think booty swing!." It's just about swinging both hips equally and pushing off with the leg in each stride, that is, if your kinetic chain isn't broken. Initially, I was frustrated and felt like my legs weren't behaving like they should. I was getting extremely sore in the left gluteal muscles and in my left quadriceps too. It seemed almost impossible to get the left gluteal muscles to work correctly. The upside was that the change of gait made it obvious which muscles needed the most strengthening. Thinking about how I used my muscles with each stride forced me to pay attention to which muscles were working and which ones were not doing their job. As soon as I stopped paying attention, willing muscle helpers were on standby to take over the job of the weak muscles. Keep in mind that your gait and muscle patterns may differ from mine. My objective here is to help you increase your body awareness.

In the chapter on hip anatomy, I mention the abductor muscles as important pelvis stabilizers that are crucial during gait. They are very important and they also influence knee and lower back function (30). However, the abductor function is just one of many components of the gait cycle. Gait is complex and involves a whole chain of muscle movements. It is beyond the scope of this book to go into great detail on the gait cycle, but I do want to cover the basics and emphasize the importance of gait analysis, because it can provide valuable information on the order in which your muscles fire and potential weaknesses you may have. If the muscle firing order is off, there may be consequences up the kinetic chain. You may even experience pain in your back and/or shoulder.

The process of gait happens in different phases. There is the stance phase, where one leg is fixed on the ground with the foot flat. While one leg is in the stance phase, the other leg is in the swing phase. Each swing phase begins with the toe lifting off the ground, when the foot is getting ready to leave the ground to swing. The swing phase ends with heel contact, or heel strike, when the heel lands on the ground. Through the processes of stance and swing, heel strike and toe off, different muscles fire with varying intensity. Three muscle groups at the hip play an important role during walking: the hip extensors, the hip flexors and the hip abductors (9).

Let's look at how the muscles fire during gait. Although there is some disagreement on the firing order (some researchers say that the gluteus maximus firing can be delayed without being abnormal, and causing lumbopelvic pain) (32), I will review the most common perception. The primary hip extensor, the gluteus maximus is slowly activated toward the end of the swing phase. By the time the heel hits the ground, entering the stance phase, gluteus maximus is strongly activated to prevent uncontrollable trunk flexion. The gluteus maximus remains active from heel contact until the middle of the stance phase (the first 30 percent of the gait cycle). The hamstrings only assist the gluteus maximus during the first 10 percent of the gait cycle (9).

The key role of the hip flexors is to bring the leg forward during the swing phase, to prepare for the next step. The primary hip flexor, the iliopsoas, becomes active before toe off to slow down the rate of the hip extension. It also helps to bring the hip into initial swing. The movement of hip flexion stays active until the end of the swing phase, but the hip flexors are only considered active for the first 50 percent of the swing. The second half of the hip flexion movement is a result of passive forward momentum and gravity. The rectus femoris muscle assists the iliopsoas. The hip abductors provide stability to the pelvis during gait and keep the pelvis from dropping while one leg is swinging (9).

There is a principle called the law of reciprocal inhibition in muscle physiology. It states that when an agonist muscle (a muscle that causes the primary motion) is stimulated, the antagonist (muscle moving a joint in the opposite direction) must be relatively inhibited. For example, if psoas (hip flexor and agonist) is activated, the gluteus maximus (a hip extensor and antagonist of psoas) has to be limited or the hip won't flex. At the same time, the antagonist activation is needed to keep the hip from flexing uncontrollably, thus it is a question of degree of facilitation and inhibition.

Osteopathy has taken the law of reciprocal inhibition a bit further by developing the tight-loose concept. This concept states that the tighter an agonist muscle becomes, the looser and weaker the antagonist muscle. For example: the tighter psoas is, the looser and weaker the gluteus maximus (33). But the hamstrings are hip extensors too, so according to the law of reciprocal inhibition wouldn't they be loose and weak? Why are the hamstrings instead commonly tight in FAI patients?

The hamstring tightness can be explained by the concept of altered reciprocal inhibition and synergistic dominance. Altered reciprocal inhibition means that there is decreased neural drive to the antagonist muscle because the agonist muscle is overactive. Consequently, when the hip flexors are overactive and tight it causes a decrease in neural drive to the gluteus maximus. If you recall from the chapter on hip anatomy, a synergist muscle assists another muscle in accomplishing a movement. The hamstrings act as synergists for gluteus maximus (34).

Synergistic dominance occurs when the main agonist is weak and not firing correctly. In our example, the hamstrings go beyond their assisting function and start taking over the role of the gluteus maximus. As synergists, the hamstrings are not supposed to be the sole hip extensors. They are only supposed to be active for the first 10 percent of the gait cycle. Taking over for gluteus maximus, they have to work too hard, and become tight and fatigued. Sometimes, people with overworked hamstrings get pain and cramps in the hamstrings and back of the knees and are put at risk for hamstring strains (34).

8.2.2 *Strengthening*

Once your gait and muscle imbalances have been properly analyzed, you can get on the right track with strengthening exercises. With my new and improved body awareness, I only started the process of strengthening the weak muscles after my physical therapy ended. Now, you might think: "What on Earth did she do at physical therapy?." I understand your question. Of course, I did lots of strengthening at physical therapy. But, I thought the physical therapy would take care of all my muscle-related problems. As it turned out, my physical therapist sees so many patients that it was hard to get one-on-one attention. If I were a million-dollar athlete, I am sure a whole entourage of well-paid health care professionals would have poured their energy into my rehabilitation. But most of us don't get the royal treatment, meaning we have to take charge and participate.

My physical therapy included quad, hamstring and gluteal strengthening. I would use the same amount of weight and the same number of repetitions for both left and right sides. Exercises were not modified to prevent muscles like the hamstrings and adductors from taking over. Indeed, I got stronger. What was weak got stronger, but what was already tight and overworked also got stronger. Trigger points got much worse in my hamstrings and adductors, to the point where much of the strengthening was next to impossible to perform because of pain. The gluteal strengthening exercises were not modified either, like they should have been in order to put the lowest possible load on the tendinitis prone iliopsoas. As a result, my muscles were allowed to keep the firing patterns they had acquired during the years of untreated FAI. After 40 visits of physical therapy for each hip I felt much of the same muscle pain that I had experienced before the surgeries. The good news was that the hip joints were feeling great — no more of that catching and locking!

Sometimes, it is hard to strengthen muscles because of pain. If you have a lot of myofascial adhesions or trigger points, you may benefit from alternating strengthening therapy with myofascial release or trigger point dry needling. If your soft tissue is too stuck, strengthening may not be effective, and soft tissue pain can persist because the muscle fibers and connective tissue need to glide properly to work. Depending on your specific gait and imbalance patterns, your physical therapist should modify — within the limits prescribed by your surgeon — your exercises to avoid overworking muscles that are already working overtime.

If your soft tissue is too stuck, strengthening may not be effective, and soft tissue pain can persist because the muscle fibers and connective tissue need to glide properly to work.

There are various muscle activation techniques (MAT) that can be employed to break undesirable muscle activation patterns during gait and strengthening (see 8.3 Additional Therapies). In addition, exercises may need to be modified to keep synergist muscles from taking over the work of agonists during strengthening. For example, if your hamstrings work too hard during hip extension, your physical therapist needs to adjust gluteal strengthening to inhibit the hamstrings (34).

In addition, leg press exercises on a leg press machine and bridge exercises can be modified to prevent the adductors from contracting too much and allow the gluteal muscles to do the work. You can put a looped Thera-Band® around your feet and push your feet outward to tension the Thera-Band at the same time as performing leg presses lying on your back on a leg press machine. This will decrease the contraction of the adductors and emphasize strengthening of the gluteal muscles. These modified exercises are just examples. Your knowledge of muscle imbalances and body awareness will put you in a position to discuss your rehabilitation with your physical therapist to further modify your exercise program to fit your needs.

8.2.3 Stretching

Your strongholds, muscles that have been overworked and taking over the work of weaker muscles may be sore, short and tight. If you work and strengthen those muscles to the same extent as the weak muscles, they will not only become stronger, but, in my personal experience, they may become even tighter too. The trigger points I had in these muscles, for example my hamstrings and adductors, only got worse. Once I had identified those muscles, I felt that I was better off leaving them be, at least temporarily, not to strengthen them, but only stretch them, get trigger point massage, dry needling and Sarapin® injections (see 8.3 Additional Therapies).

During physical therapy, I was never told to stretch the hamstrings. However, once I did my gait analysis and consciously worked to change the way I walk, I realized that the hamstrings had been completely overused. They now needed some love. I would do the classic hamstring stretch where you lie on your back, bring up one leg straight and wrap a towel or a sheet around your flexed foot. My hamstrings were actually so tight and full of trigger points that the towel stretch barely made a dent in the tightness. I then progressed to the doorway stretch where one leg goes up against a wall, and the other leg lies on the floor through a doorway. That stretch can be quite intense, and I ended up straining my hamstrings somewhat in trying to get them relaxed. What ultimately helped the most was the Sarapin® injected into the hamstring trigger points (see 8.3.5 Sarapin).

While stretching is helpful to most people, you can also do too much. For the longest time, before my FAI diagnosis, I had received well-intended advice from friends and medical professionals alike. The most common piece of advice was "do some yoga: yoga is great; do some stretching." I would try — and fail miserably. Stretching certain ways and yoga made the FAI pain worse. In addition, for a person with a fair amount of joint hypermobility, stretching just isn't always the right solution.

In general, physical therapists love to stretch the iliopsoas muscle. Unfortunately, my psoas doesn't love to be stretched. The commonly used Thomas stretch, where you let one leg dangle off the table, stabilizing yourself with your core and bring the other leg flexed toward your chest, does not sit well with me. I have lost count of the number of physical therapists who wanted me to stretch iliopsoas in this or other ways before the hip arthroscopies — and it would always set off pain. In the process of being diagnosed with FAI, I learned that the psoas muscle is a typical culprit for FAI patients, and sometimes remains a source of pain well after the FAI surgeries. On a side note, the Thomas stretch actually involves two extremes in one stretch: full hip extension for the dangling leg and full hip flexion for the other leg.

There may be some scientific evidence that physical therapists and body workers in general, may be too psoas-stretch-happy. Using a biomechanical model of the hip joint, a researcher looked at the influence of hip position and muscle function during movements and exercises over the course of four studies. In essence, the result of the studies was that anterior hip force, which is associated with anterior hip pain and labral tears, increased most with the greatest degree of hip extension. The study also found that, even when optimal force was created, hip extension was related to anterior hip force whereas hip flexion was not. Optimal force occurs when gluteus maximus produces the maximal force for hip extension, instead of other muscles taking up the slack, and when iliopsoas produces the maximum force for hip flexion. One of the points the researcher made is that hip extension should be minimized. Ultimately, it means that if the hip flexors aren't tight, don't stretch them by default (35).

After my FAI surgeries I made a 100 percent effort to follow the physical therapy program. Because I knew that my surgeon had released my psoas during the surgery, I thought it would be beneficial to stretch this muscle like the post-surgical physical therapy program prescribed. Not so. Sure, my psoas got more and more flexible doing the Thomas stretch and I definitely reached a point of great flexibility of the psoas, but pain would follow every time. At some point during the rehabilitation program, my physical therapist and I just decided to scrap it and not aggravate the pain.

As I am writing this, I received a new diagnosis that may or may not explain the post-surgical difficulties with the iliopsoas stretch — hidden hernias, both inguinal and femoral. The future will tell if the hip flexors are actually tight and painful or if the pain occurred as a result of hernias. No matter what the cause, we need to listen to our bodies. If something consistently hurts, there is an underlying cause. Pain is just a symptom.

Does pain with the Thomas-stretch mean that the iliopsoas muscle is not important and should not be stretched? Not necessarily. I found that both gentle release of the psoas during therapeutic massage and dry needling of this muscle were helpful techniques for keeping the psoas happy without the aggravating pain.

Stretching the piriformis muscle in the buttock is also one of those standard recipes physical therapists serve if you have sacroiliac pain or piriformis syndrome. The question is, do you actually have true sacroiliac pain or do you have muscle pain in the buttocks? A diagnostic sacroiliac joint injection will give you the answer. Personally, I have never noted a benefit from stretching the piriformis. However, it did hurt my hips before the surgeries. Both psoas and piriformis can also be released with a gentle technique called body rolling (see 8.3.2 Body Rolling).

8.3 Additional Therapies

There are some additional therapies that can assist with the rehabilitation from surgery to treat FAI. Maybe you have finished your physical therapy program, and are looking for alternate ways of getting better. Or you may still be doing physical therapy, but feel that it is not quite doing the trick. Just because your insurance company won't cover any more physical therapy, or you've finished your prescribed program, doesn't mean you can't keep getting better. It's common to continue improving over a long period of time after FAI surgery (6). In addition to doing exercises that work for you, there are some alternative therapies you can try to help with soft tissue pain, trigger points and remaining muscle imbalances. In the following section, I will explore some therapies I have tried or would have liked to try.

8.3.1 Therapeutic Massage

I consider myself a lucky woman to have a friend who is also an excellent massage therapist. Well into the recovery from my left hip arthroscopy (my second hip surgery), I started getting therapeutic massage almost every week. The bodywork my friend does is not your typical relaxing spa massage. In fact, it's torturous at times, like when she does deep work on the psoas, adductors and gluteal muscles.

Knowing when to get a post-operative massage can be a bit complicated. The timing depends on the type of surgery, how deep the surgery was, and how big the incision is. Everybody is unique and heals at different rates, but there are general guidelines to follow. First, ask your doctor and get his/her approval before getting massage. For a minor surgery with a smaller incision, the area can be avoided for the first few days or weeks and the rest of the body can be massaged. For major surgery, the time limit before you can receive a massage will be six to twelve weeks (36).

Massage therapy helps healing in four stages: pain relief, adhesion reduction, muscle balancing, and maintenance. During the first few massage sessions after an injury or surgery, the goal is to reduce tension and relieve pain. Once pain is reduced, the underlying cause can be addressed to correct the problem and free up adhesions and scar tissue. Massage can strengthen surrounding tissues so they can provide more balanced support once the injury has healed. Having regular maintenance massages can help prevent injury and speed up the healing process. It is also important to re-educate your muscles to provide correct posture and movement in addition to receiving massages (36) .

Therapeutic massage can involve various modalities, one being massage cupping. Massage cups originate with Chinese medicine, where fire was used to create a vacuum in a glass cup. The modern version of massage cupping uses plastic/rubber cups to create a vacuum seal on the body. When used during massage, the cups may be moved in different patterns across the body to loosen adhesions and lift connective tissue. The intensity can be adjusted. If you have a lot of adhesions, massage cupping can feel intense at first, but you will feel great afterward. Massage sessions can also involve active release stretches for muscles like the iliopsoas muscle.

My massage therapist sometimes uses little balls called t spheres® to work and release trigger points in different areas. I sometimes use the t spheres® on myself to rub out an area or just sit or lie on them where I feel a trigger point. Massage therapists have different specializations. Some therapists have taken training in a lot of different techniques, like neuromuscular and craniosacral therapy, while others only do Swedish and deep tissue massage. You can experiment with different types of massage. Always make sure that you stay within the limits of the surgeon's restrictions when you get massaged after surgery.

8.3.2 *Body Rolling*

My massage therapist not only introduced me to massage, but also to body or ball rolling. The principles of ball rolling exist in similar ways under several names. I have come to be familiar with Yamuna® Body Rolling because it was a technique I tried long before I was diagnosed with FAI. Using balls of varying sizes made of a sturdy yet flexible material, body rolling helps you create space between muscle and bone, allowing for correct alignment. The idea is to let the body's circuit board fire in the logical and correct order (37).

Once you have performed a body rolling routine on one side of your body, you'll feel a big difference compared to the untreated side. The muscles will feel elongated. For FAI patients, body rolling can be helpful, because the ball gives you the opportunity to lengthen the short hip rotators and work the muscles that are otherwise hard to get to. One of the ball rolling routines involves starting with the ball under the ischial tuberosity, rolling down onto the muscle tendons, cross fibering (moving horizontally from one side of the leg to the other) to separate adductor magnus and the hamstrings, and break up adhesions. The routine then moves back onto the ischial tuberosity and incrementally rolls out the short hip rotators, gluteus maximus, minimus and medius as well as tensor fasciae latae.

There are many different routines for various body parts. Ball rolling is not pain free. The pressure on certain muscles and spots may feel quite intense, but if you can endure you can eventually feel better. To find a certified Yamuna body rolling instructor you can visit www.yamunabodyrolling.com. You can also buy instructional DVDs, books and balls and just go at it yourself.

8.3.3 *Active Release Techniques*

Having tried Active Release Techniques® (ART) I have to disagree slightly with the official description of ART. On the ART website you can read that ART is a patented soft tissue system/movement based massage technique that treats problems with muscles, tendons, ligaments, fascia and nerves (Active Release Techniques 2010). The ART treatments I received didn't resemble massage. Deep massage can hurt but ART put me in tears. To me, ART is better described as forceful stretching with applied pressure than as massage. ART treatments start an inflammatory process in the soft tissues. I am aware that many FAI patients who have tried ART post-surgically have experienced good results, but there are also patient anecdotes telling a different story, for whom ART caused a new or worse pain.

My flirtation with ART was short-lived because it was quite obvious that it did me more harm than good. Four months after my few ART treatments, I am still in worse pain than I was before the treatments. Nonetheless, I still think ART can work for many in helping to break up adhesions from muscle overuse. Based on my experience with ART and that of other patients, ART needs to be approached with a bit of caution. As a non-scientific explanation, I think it's possible for ART practitioners to give some people's soft tissue more than it can handle and cause more than the intended healthy inflammation. Not all connective tissue is the same and does not respond to treatment in the same way.

Still, for some patients, ART can be a good therapy to try. Make sure the ART provider really listens to you in order to find the treatment level that works for you. Too much pressure and too much stretching may not work and possibly make you worse. You can find certified ART practitioners at www.activerelease.com. In my geographic area, there are hardly any physical therapists who are certified in ART, but quite a few chiropractors. Based on personal my experience with chiropractic over the course of eight years, having seen about six different providers, given the choice between a physical therapist and a chiropractor I would always go for a physical therapist. Chiropractors have a different overall philosophy than physical therapists, and many of them just get itchy adjustment fingers whenever they see a sacroiliac joint. Adjustments are not always beneficial.

8.3.4 *Muscle Activation Techniques*

Some FAI patients have had success restoring muscle balance by means of Muscle Activation Techniques® (MAT), a system designed to evaluate and treat muscular imbalances. According to the founder of MAT, the method consists of basic concepts from physiology and biomechanics that have been converted to a systematic approach. The goal is to determine whether or not specific muscles supporting a joint have the necessary input from the body's nervous system to perform their function. If a muscle does not have the needed input, it will not able to perform its function efficiently (38).

Through Muscle Activation Techniques, muscles with improper neurological connections are identified and jumpstarted, allowing them to stabilize the joints and reduce joint stress. The ultimate goal is for the body to become more efficient. The related aches and pains are then deterred (38). MAT-certified providers may be found on the website, www.muscleactivation.com. Had there been a practitioner in my area, I'm sure I would have tried MAT.

8.3.5 *Sarapin*

One year after my first surgery that I ran into a physiatrist (PMR doctor) at a birthday party. We struck up a conversation and I ended up seeing him in his office, where he told me about Sarapin®, a plant substance I wish now I'd heard about much earlier. No physician I had seen over the years — and that's not a small number — had ever told me about Sarapin. With a healthy dose of skepticism I went home and researched Sarapin before going back and asking to try it. Sarapin is a liquid solution derived from the pitcher plant that has been shown to relieve pain and break up trigger points. By now, I have received Sarapin injections in my hamstrings, adductors and calf muscles, back and shoulder muscles and it helps a lot with muscle pain and trigger points. You can expect to be sore from the injections on the day of, but it dissipates, as does the pain.

One reason you might never have heard of Sarapin is that it's not a drug. That means that pharmaceutical companies neither sell nor market Sarapin, and it may not even reach your doctor's office. If you still have a lot of myofascial pain and trigger points after hip surgery, or in general, it is worth calling around to see if a doctor in your area does Sarapin injections. I found these injections well worth the price of admission.

8.4 How Long to Wait between Hip Surgeries

Different surgeons have different opinions on how long to wait between surgeries. At first, I was told to wait a minimum of six weeks between surgeries. I felt that six weeks would be too soon. Continuing my physical therapy all the way up to surgery number two, I waited three months between surgeries. Could I have done the second surgery sooner? Yes, but not by much. For me, three months was about right, but that's not necessarily the golden number for everyone.

According to Dr. Hanson of Henderson, Nevada, an unpublished study conducted by Dr. Philippon at the Steadman Philippon Research Institute shows no significant difference in terms of outcome when waiting a longer or shorter time between surgeries. Dr. Hanson thinks it comes down to having a good leg to stand on. "You want to have your first surgery far enough through the post-operative period that you have good strength in your muscles and are able to stabilize and protect the hip joint without causing a hip flexor tendinitis or other irritation because you are now non-weight-bearing on the other side." (6)

9 INJURIES SECONDARY TO HIP IMPINGEMENT

As previously discussed, patients with hip impingement and tears of the labrum often develop muscle imbalances and pain that is secondary to the actual problem, the hip. The root cause being the mechanical alterations in the hip, a person with hip impingement may not only develop muscle imbalances, but also injuries due to muscle compensation. A 2007 study on the clinical presentation of FAI concluded that 92 percent of the 301 patients in the study reported difficulty during prolonged participation in sports. In order to continue in their sports, 71 percent of the patients had to modify their technique (3). When you modify your technique and allow your body to compensate for the body parts that are not able to perform their job you can develop both compensatory hip pain and compensatory injuries.

Most commonly, patients with FAI have limited internal hip rotation and flexion because of the bone abnormalities. When there is a mismatch between the hip motion required for normal function and the motion possible in our bodies, a compensatory increase in motion may be provided by the lumbar spine, sacroiliac (SI) joint and pubic symphysis. The dynamic muscle force across the pelvis may occur with altered motion and result in excessive strain at these joints and the muscles that attach to them. In some patients, restoring the normal motion at the hip joint is enough to normalize the joint mechanics (39). Sometimes, however, FAI surgery is not enough to reverse injuries secondary to FAI, so those need to be addressed separately. In the following, I will explore some of the secondary injury patterns commonly seen with FAI.

9.1 Osteitis Pubis

If you recall from the chapter on basic hip anatomy, the left and the right sides of the pubic bone are connected in the middle by a cartilage disc, the pubic symphysis joint. Osteitis pubis is a condition of diffuse pain, instability, inflammation and bony changes at that joint. Sports that require a lot of twisting, kicking and turning, like soccer, hockey and American football, but also distance running, are associated with osteitis pubis. The pain can be on one or both sides. The adductor muscles that attach on the pubic bone are often involved with this injury. Pain can be reproduced if the doctor palpates the pubic symphysis joint or performs resisted hip adduction. That is, you try to squeeze your legs together and the doctor holds his/her arms between your legs giving providing resistance (39).

The onset of osteitis pubis is mostly gradual. If x-rays are obtained during the acute phase, the films often read as normal. When the injury becomes chronic, x-rays may show sclerosis (hardening of tissue sometimes due to inflammation, or an increase of connective tissue), cystic changes or widening of the joint space. An MRI is not always helpful in diagnosing osteitis pubis, but it may show excessive fluid in the joint because of inflammation. As with most sports injuries, treatment is initially conservative consisting of anti-inflammatory medications and physical therapy including hip range of motion therapy. Sometimes, the doctor will inject the pubic symphysis with a steroid, both for diagnosis and treatment. If all non-surgical measures fail, there are various surgical options, including endoscopic placement of mesh behind the joint or open surgery with joint fixation by means of plates. Most seem to bring relief of varying degrees to a majority of patients, but none seem to have more than an 88 percent success rate (39).

9.2 Athletic Pubalgia

If you have never heard of athletic pubalgia, you might have heard of sports hernia. Some doctors oppose the term sports hernia, because there is not much physical similarity to a traditional hernia, but many patients and doctors still use this term. After all, what's easier to say: athletic pubalgia or sports hernia? If patients and doctors want this injury to become more widely recognized and correctly diagnosed, then maybe using the term athletic pubalgia makes sense, because it won't be confused with a regular hernia.

So what is athletic pubalgia? There is no one answer to that question, since the specific injury can vary. Athletic pubalgia is a set of pelvic injuries involving the abdominal and pelvic musculature outside the ball-and-socket hip joint and on both sides of the pubic symphysis joint (40). Variations may include tearing of the rectus abdominis (the "six pack" muscle), internal and external oblique muscles. Injury of the inguinal ligament (Gilmore's groin) may be involved (39). In addition, adductor tendons often cause pain, whether they have suffered tearing, are chronically tight or have tendinitis (41).

One type of athletic pubalgia occurs when the muscles or tendons in a thin region of the abdominal wall are weakened. Once overexerted, a muscle tear occurs inside what is called the groin, although the term groin is quite unspecific. The overexertion of the abdominals occurs, because they are fighting a losing battle with the adductor muscles of the hip. The oblique muscles attach at the pubis. When they contract, they pull up on the pubis as the trunk flexes and rotates. Adductor muscles also attach at the pubis; they pull on the pelvis from below as they work to move the thighbone toward or past the middle of the body. When both oblique muscles and adductor muscles contract at the same time, a tug-of-war of the pelvis ensues. Because athletes tend to focus on strengthening the lower body more than the trunk, the adductor muscles are typically stronger. As a result the weaker oblique muscles tear (42).

Another type of tearing may occur at the lower attachments of the rectus abdominis. Some literature indicates that this kind of tearing is easier to detect on MRIs with fairly high sensitivity (41). Small tears in the oblique muscles don't seem to show up on MRIs nearly as often, making it frustrating for those who suffer from this injury. A specialized physical exam and a history of the onset and the symptoms become very important in diagnosing such tears (42).

Once athletic pubalgia has occurred, pain typically develops gradually as activity increases and gets better with rest. Patients often complain of pain that radiates into the adductor muscles, perineum (the area between anus and scrotum in men and the vulva in women), rectus abdominis or testicles. The symptoms typically get worse with sit-ups, kicking, running, coughing and sneezing (41). When medical literature started reporting on athletic pubalgia, reports mainly concerned males. Experts increasingly recognize today that athletic pubalgia occurs in women as well (40). Why wouldn't it? There are probably just fewer female professional athletes and consequently fewer study subjects.

If conservative treatment, consisting of rest from aggravating activities combined with specific core and hip strengthening and anti-inflammatory medications fails, surgery may be warranted. Some doctors use the laparoscopic method and use mesh to repair and support the muscles. Other doctors prefer a small open incision to better be able to see all structures that may need repair and perform a classic tissue repair with sutures. Both types of surgery have their advantages and disadvantages, and both types can have good outcomes. Mesh causes chronic pain in some patients, but an open incision gone wrong can cause problems too.

9.3 Muscle Injury

A number of muscle injuries are associated with FAI. The adductor longus works with the abdominal muscles to stabilize the pelvis during activity, making it prone to injury. In addition to a physical exam that reveals tenderness at the adductor attachments on the pubis and pain with passive stretching, an MRI might show increased fluid signal confirming an adductor strain.

The combination of a labral tear, adductor strain and a rectus abdominis strain is so common in athletes that it has been coined the "sports hip triad." FAI is believed to intensify muscles injuries around the pelvis. Hamstring tendinitis, rectus femoris (hip flexor) avulsions, psoas tendinitis and abductor strains (gluteus medius and minimus) are also causes of groin pain commonly associated with FAI, but there is no scientific proof so far that FAI is the cause of those injuries (39).

In most cases, the treatment of muscle injuries is non-surgical and consists of the usual rest, ice, physical therapy and range of motion exercises. It is common to inject the adductor attachments with steroid to calm down inflammation. Sometimes, surgery is warranted to repair muscle tears or release shortened tendons, like the iliopsoas and the adductor longus tendons.

9.4 Posterior Hip Subluxation

Although posterior subluxation in the hip isn't something that happens to most of us, it is worth mentioning, because it is often misdiagnosed as a muscle strain or a sprain. Most often the injury occurs when an athlete falls on the hip while it is flexed and adducted. The fall could happen while playing American football or soccer, but also in sports like gymnastics or just jogging or biking. The injury may also occur without trauma or with just minimal trauma.

Lax ligaments of the hip capsule or abnormal bone shapes of the hip joint can predispose a person to hip instability. Painful limitation of hip motion and pain in the hip even when resting should raise a red flag (39).

When posterior subluxation is present, a CT scan, MRI or x-ray will show the typical fracture of the back wall of the hip socket, likely also a posterior labral tear and it may show bleeding in the joint as well as ligament disruption. Sometimes, a labral tear in the front of the hip joint will also occur, which may be caused by the crush injury secondary to underlying FAI with CAM lesions. Treatment of posterior subluxation is ultimately surgery, but the protocol varies from institution to institution, as does the timing of the treatment. The traction used during arthroscopic surgery as well as leakage of fluid because of injury to the hip capsule is a concern during the acute phase of the injury. Therefore, some doctors choose to delay surgery for at least six weeks after an injury. The decision to not delay surgery may depend on if there is a large loose body or tear of the cartilage that covers the end of a bone. Unfortunately, an active return to sports is not always possible after a posterior subluxation injury. If the hip joint develops a condition where bone tissue dies because of a lack of blood supply (osteonecrosis), sports may cause the hip joint to collapse and degenerate (39).

9.5 Lumbar Spine

While lumbar spine problems and their relationship to FAI have not yet been proven in studies (6), some physicians believe that the altered biomechanics caused by FAI increase the strain placed on the lower back. Their thinking is that when the motion of one half of the pelvis is limited, the lower back may be required to act as a source of motion for the leg on that side. As a result, various stress reactions of the facet joints of the spine may occur and cause pain. Other sources of pain, like referred pain from the spine, disc pain and deformities of the spine, have to be ruled out (39). Decreased internal rotation range of motion in the hip has been linked to lower back problems in tennis players (43).

9.6 Upper Body Stress

Dr. Bryan Kelly, an FAI and sports injury specialist at the Hospital for Special Surgery in New York, has presented study results showing that FAI not only affects the lower part of our bodies, but also the upper body. The study showed that FAI may alter the chain of movement (kinetic chain) all the way up to the shoulder (43). As is often the case, the focus of the study was on athletes, but why wouldn't its conclusions apply to FAI sufferers who are not professional athletes?

The study subjects were 34 baseball and lacrosse athletes with abnormal mechanics caused by FAI and laxity. They all underwent arthroscopic surgery to treat FAI and labral tears. The results were that their Harris hip scores improved from 70 to 92, and mechanical overload of the hip could be the cause of weakening in the athletes' sports performances. After surgery, all but one athlete went back to pre-injury levels of sports participation (44).

Presenting the research, Dr. Kelly explained how hip deformities may lead to abnormal movement patterns in the torso and upper extremity, with injuries of the upper body parts resulting from the stress placed on the torso, shoulder and elbow. The reasoning is that the lower extremity is important for generating forward momentum when throwing. If there is decreased strength, restricted range of motion, pain or apprehension in the hips, the throwing athlete cannot properly generate torque from the pelvis and lower legs. S/he is not able to use the optimal stride distance and lead-leg foot placement. Often, hip disease, like FAI, can be associated with decreased hip abductor strength. If the muscles around the hip are not working properly, there may be increased stress on shoulder and elbow. A loss of normal hip motion may also require compensation that can lead to problems in the torso and upper extremities (43).

10 PREGNANCY AND HIP IMPINGEMENT

Obviously, we each have to make our own decision about getting pregnant while dealing with untreated FAI and labral tears. There is no scientific literature on FAI and pregnancy. Based on numerous personal stories, women have very different experiences with FAI during pregnancy. It is common for women to have hip pain due to FAI during pregnancy, but many may be undiagnosed at that point.

Some women actually report feeling better during pregnancy and sometimes for a while after pregnancy. One explanation for this improvement could be that the hormone relaxin, released in a woman's body to prepare for childbirth, helps relax and soften joints and muscles. If you normally have a restricted range of motion from FAI, the relaxin released during pregnancy could work to your advantage. However, if you were slightly hypermobile before pregnancy, with a range of motion exceeding the ordinary, the relaxin could lead to even more mobility and joint instability.

No one knows for sure why some female FAI sufferers report having less pain during pregnancy and there are also women who have hip impingement and suffer tremendous pain during pregnancy. Pregnancy can be a rough bodily state for women in general, but if you have FAI and labral tears pregnancy will add weight onto hip joints that are already malfunctioning.

Even if you read a million patient testimonials and learn all the facts about labral tears, FAI and pregnancy, the decision still has to be yours. A lot of undiagnosed women become pregnant and survive pregnancy. The question is, with what level of pain. It is possible that pregnancy and childbirth will accelerate and aggravate the hip deterioration and pain. The way vaginal deliveries are done in most hospitals, with legs abducted and externally rotated in stirrups, puts the woman into a poor position for impinged hip joints. A fair number of labral tears, with or without FAI as their root cause, occur during childbirth (45).

We have to consider more than one issue when deciding on having children. It becomes an equation of life-impacting factors like age, health insurance, employment, potentially other illnesses and of course how much moms and dads want a baby. Sometimes babies just happen. Despite the pain from FAI and whatever else life throws at us, we love them unconditionally.

10.1 Personal Experiences with Pregnancy and Hip Impingement

Unfortunately, I belonged to the group of women who suffered with a lot of pain through pregnancy. Because no doctor could find anything wrong with me, my husband and I eventually decided to go for it. I was 32 at the time, and felt that time was running away from me. It wasn't until our son was a little over two that I finally received the diagnosis of hip impingement. Had I received this diagnosis earlier, my decision would have been to treat the hip impingement first and postpone pregnancy.

My pain increased during pregnancy, and stayed at a higher level after pregnancy than before. I have a certain amount of hypermobility, which also increased as pregnancy progressed. My pain was so bad that I'd have to stop walking in the middle of a step. Despite only putting on a normal amount of weight, I was in a rough state. At six months gestation, I started a physical therapy program that helped put me back together enough so I could at least function. Luckily for me, this was our first baby, and I had the luxury of not having any major obligations at the time. I was already not working a full-time job, and could decide to work as my condition allowed. I did work a little all the way to the end, but at least the pressure was off.

Before my husband and I found out that our baby was breech (buttocks down instead of head down), I had repeatedly told my OB that I didn't think I could handle delivering with my legs in stirrups because my hips would lock. He disregarded all of my concerns because, first, I had no diagnosis or proof to lean on, and, second, most women in America don't decide how to deliver a baby, their doctors do. Would the damage to my hips have been made even worse with a normal delivery? Since I had a c-section I won't know the answer, but I do know this: I don't ever want another c-section and I will go to great lengths to have a VBAC (vaginal birth after cesarean) should we be so lucky to have another child.

After delivery, my body was is in rather poor shape. Recovering from a c-section as well as battling hip, groin and buttock pain — oh, then there was the impinged shoulder — I seriously struggled with everyday (baby) tasks. Before pregnancy, I never realized how much bending, carrying and laundry I would have to do with a baby — an endless list of hip and back unfriendly tasks. I had trouble carrying the car seat, lifting strollers, carrying a baby who got heavier each day, and eventually chasing a sprinting toddler and cleaning up spills from the floor.

After a while we hired help, but not exactly a full-time nanny and housekeeper. Be happy about any help you can get! If someone comes over to look at the baby and you are struggling, ask them to throw in a load of laundry or help you empty the dishwasher. If you pay someone, obviously you can expect more help than if a friend comes over to socialize. Do line up help! If my husband and I had known what to expect, we would have planned differently for the baby's arrival.

Then there is the issue of having surgeries when you have a young child. Open or not, hip surgeries are not easy. If I had had the choice of getting pregnant on purpose with untreated FAI or first having the FAI surgeries, I would have fixed the hips first. But God works in mysterious ways, and we have a lot to be grateful for.

11 BE THE ENTREPRENEURIAL PATIENT

If you have been a consumer of health care for a while, either trying to get a diagnosis for your pain or dealing with some type of chronic health issue, you have probably encountered the many hurdles and challenges of the American health care system. While there are some excellent doctors and some well-run practices and hospitals, there are quite a few that don't operate smoothly or produce good outcomes.

As the Entrepreneurial Patient you might not be able to fix the system, but by taking some rather simple, systematic steps you can get insurance authorizations, diagnostic tests and care more quickly. Since I have already stepped on many landmines, you can learn from and take advantage of my mistakes. Educating yourself on conditions like FAI, you can find an excellent doctor and get the right and necessary tests for an accurate diagnosis. Prevention is better than fighting a fire. So, if you want faster results, you have be pro-active and work smarter, not necessarily harder.

This book about the Entrepreneurial Patient covers topics that may benefit hip impingement patients. For a wider spectrum of health insurance and health care topics, look for new books in the series *The Entrepreneurial Patient.*

11.1 Ideas for Communicating with Your Doctor

Have you ever walked out of a doctor's office disappointed by how your appointment went? Or have you ever gotten into your car just to remember too late what you wanted to ask the doctor? I certainly have in the past. But those days are over now. Somewhere along the way, I laid down some ground rules for myself to determine how I could get the most out of every appointment. There have been some doctors, however, with whom I knew almost immediately that it wasn't worth spending my time. In those cases I walked out fairly quickly and sucked up the co-pay. Here is the format I normally follow before and during a doctor's appointment.

> *Prepare for an important doctor's appointment like you would for a business meeting. Research online, always checking on the credibility of your sources. Some doctors are not thrilled with patients who bring their own ideas and research, but research allows you to ask relevant questions. You have the right to be taken seriously when you bring up thoughts, questions and treatment ideas that your doctor wasn't considering. Your doctor doesn't need to agree with you, but shouldn't dismiss you.*
>
> *Bring your agenda. Make a list ahead of your doctor's appointment with discussion points, questions, thoughts, research and ideas.*

Be ready to give the doctor important information and correct data about yourself. He or she usually does not have a lot of time to look at your medical records from other medical providers, so you have to connect the dots. Make sure you bring records, imaging films and/or CDs.

If your doctor doesn't listen to you, take control of the conversation. Whenever I feel that a doctor is trying to run me over, I interrupt. Sometimes that's the only way to get your point across. If he or she is still not listening, switch doctors!

Take notes, especially if a topic is new to you. It's annoying to come home ready to conduct more research when you can't remember the name of a procedure or test. If you are going to see several doctors, it is helpful to go through the notes from other doctor's visits as you prepare for a new appointment.

If your doctor speaks Latin and you don't, ask for a translation: "Excuse me, what does synovium mean?"

Get your imaging reports before your follow up appointment. It's a good idea to have a copy of your imaging report before you go to the doctor's office for a follow-up appointment. I like to read the report and research the results. If I don't have time to do the research before I go to the appointment, I at least make a note to ask the doctor about anything I don't understand.

If possible, learn some basic anatomy. You don't need to know everything, but a basic understanding can improve doctor-patient communication. Second-hand anatomy books are available online for a discounted price and if you live in a city with a university, the university library is always a good resource.

11.2 Insurance

Hopefully, you have good medical insurance, but even if you have great health coverage, there are plenty of obstacles you can run into during your medical quest. There are measures you can take to increase your odds of success when dealing with your insurance company. Great strides were made regarding FAI in 2011. To predict and analyze every reader's health insurance plan would be impossible. My experiences are based on the plans I have been enrolled in and information from other patients. In addition, I will share general advice about dealing with health insurance companies.

11.2.1 General Advice Talking to Your Health Insurer

Have you ever felt like your insurance company is giving you the run-around? Sometimes they won't be able to answer your questions, give you contradicting answers, transfer you around or put you in a catch 22. As the Entrepreneurial Patient you won't be able to completely avoid these situations, but you can learn how to navigate them more quickly. There will still be frustrations, but you will know what to do.

Tip No. 1: Get a reference number

Whether the issue is one of payment, pre-authorization or eligibility, I follow a few simple rules when I call my insurance company. First of all, I get out my notepad and pen. Once I have a representative on the line I, ask for his or her ID number or a call reference number. I do this first, before I forget. If there is an ongoing issue that is going to require several phone calls, it is helpful to have a call reference number. The next time you call the company, the representative who picks up your call will be able to retrieve the notes taken by the previous representative. Of course, it is annoying that you can't talk to the same person again, but that's how the system works, so work within it!

Tip No. 2: Take notes

For example, Ruthie Representative tells you that you do not need pre-authorization for a certain procedure or test. You will want to make note of whom you spoke with (name and ID number), call reference number, what day and time you called and what information you were given. If, in the future, it turns out that Ruthie Representative gave you incorrect information, and you are suffering the consequences in the form of non-coverage or a bill, you will be glad to have your notes to lean on when you write or call about your problem.

Tip No. 3: Dig for information

How many times have you heard the empty phrase: "Thanks for calling X. Have I answered all your questions today?" You will be asked this question, even if you just had an unsatisfactory conversation with an insurance representative who failed to properly answer your questions. No matter how inflexible the phone representative is, try to ask many questions and dig deeper.

For example, if you ask a question about eligibility for a specific procedure, the representative is likely to go straight to the reference material and read sections about your benefits plan. Most often, s/he doesn't actually know more about your plan than what s/he's reading to you, because the same representative probably takes calls from members of many different plans offered by the same insurance company. So when you ask questions about meeting specific criteria, you may only get answers like "medical necessity has to be proven" or "I am not medically trained." The representative will not be able to give you a CPT (Current Procedural Terminology) code or look up a procedure by name.

I am not medically trained either, but I know how to do research. So after I have given the representative a CPT code and confirmed that the CPT code stands for the procedure I am asking about, I search for the insurance company's name, the CPT code or procedure name, and the words coverage policy. Usually, I immediately find the relevant coverage policy. There is one caveat, however; a specific benefits plan may present an exclusion to a coverage policy that otherwise applies to all of an insurance company's customers.

Tip No. 4: Work your way up the food chain

Sometimes, if I need more detailed information directly from the insurance company, I request to speak to a supervisor. If I'm told that the supervisor won't know more than the representative, I'm usually even more convinced that I should speak to a supervisor. I usually say something like: "Well, you say your supervisor won't be able to help me, but I asked you about the specific reasons for a denial (or whatever the issue is), and you weren't able to answer. There has to be someone at your company who can answer that question. I will start with your supervisor. Can you please connect me now? Thanks so much for your help." This usually works. Sometimes the supervisor will provide information that contradicts what the representative said. Other times the supervisor doesn't know the answer to your question either. That's when you walk up the food chain and get the next manager up the chain on the phone. Keep on going until you have gathered as much information as possible!

Tip No. 5: Double check

If the information you received from a customer service representative seems too good to be true, call again and get someone else on the phone. If you get the same answer from more than one person, then maybe the good information is actually true — it does happen. But it also happens that customers receive conflicting answers to the same question. In that case, I would call a few more times talk to different representatives to see what seems like the correct answer to my question because the quality level among insurance company representatives seems to vary.

11.2.2 Pre-Authorizations, Denials and Appeals

Health care can be stressful for patients. After consulting with your doctors, you have to make the final call on whether to undergo a procedure or not. Or, don't we? Sometimes, your health insurance company adds a layer of complexity to your decision-making by putting obstacles in your way during the pre-authorization process. Other times, the authorization process is smooth. In fact, some insurance plans (especially PPO plans) do not even require pre-authorization for certain outpatient procedures or diagnostic tests. But quite often, there is a hang-up that may cause a delay in treatment.

My current insurance company almost routinely requests additional clinical information from the medical provider for advanced imaging, but does not even pre-authorize outpatient surgery or injections. It doesn't seem to matter whether the information they request has already been submitted or not; they ask for it anyway. It has even happened that they request additional information for a procedure to then deny it all together citing that the procedure is explicitly excluded in the benefits plan. For patients, the process of pre-authorization can be both confusing and frustrating. In the following section, I will explore some strategies and tactics that will give you the upper hand.

Tip No. 1: Prevent the denial

The best thing you can do to prevent a denial is to research the applicable coverage policy from your insurance company. In many cases, you can find the coverage policy online just by typing your insurer's name and the procedure or the CPT code into an Internet search engine (example: cigna cpt code hip arthroscopy). Understanding what requirements your insurance company has for covering a certain procedure or test, you will be able to give your doctor's office useful insight into the clinical information your insurance company requires.

For example, your doctor may suggest a lumbar spine MRI for you. You may read the coverage policy for a lumbar spine MRI and find out that the insurance company requires three months of relevant physical therapy with continuing or worsening pain to cover the imaging study. If you have done three months of physical therapy, that information should be detailed, and submitted to the insurance company with the initial request for pre-authorization. If you have not done three months of physical therapy, there may be other clinical findings that indicate you should get a lumbar spine MRI if you don't meet the criteria as stated in the coverage position.

In the specific instance of the lumbar MRI request as described above, an example of additional clinical findings may be that you previously had a pelvis MRI done. A pelvis MRI typically doesn't show the lumbar spine in detail. If the pelvis MRI indicates an abnormal fluid signal at, let's say, L-5/S-1, and if that finding is documented somewhere, by a radiologist or even a different physician who reviewed the films, then that clinical information needs to be submitted with the original request.

Work with your doctor's authorization staff to submit as much relevant clinical information as possible from the very beginning. That will increase your chances of getting approved without hang-ups. In addition to reviewing the coverage policy and understanding the criteria for coverage, ask questions to understand how your physician's office performs the insurance submissions. Sometimes I get in touch with the authorization representative at the doctor's office to make sure we are on the same page. About half of the time, that person had not received all the details, and I've saved all of us a lot of time by providing additional information, like copies of past studies, physical therapy records or medical records directly to the person who submits the request.

Tip No. 2: Make sure basics are covered

Before your doctor's office submits a request, make sure you have fulfilled basic requirements like getting a new x-ray done before requesting an MRI. Regarding imaging of the hips, insurance companies often want to see that an x-ray was obtained before advanced imaging can be approved. Even though that doesn't make sense when both you and your doctor know that what you need to see is the labrum, just make sure the record of an x-ray is submitted with the original request. By covering the basics, you can prevent denials and save yourself time and annoyance.

Tip No. 3: Understand how your insurance company operates

Submitting the right clinical information with a request for pre-authorization can prevent a denial, but sometimes, the response to the request is delayed or the request is denied despite careful preparation. If an authorization has taken more than a week — the time frame varies from company to company — I usually call the insurance or third-party authorization company and check the status of the request. Insurers have different ways of processing requests. Some companies don't even process their own authorizations for certain procedures, but have contracted with third-party authorization companies to perform all case reviews, especially for advanced imaging tests like CT and MRIs.

If you have been informed of a denial and call your insurance company, don't be surprised if they tell you to call Authorization Company XYZ. They should always send you a written notification of denial or approval, but sometimes you find out the results from your doctor's office before the letter makes it to your mailbox. My experience from calls inquiring about a status request is that the representative you first encounter will tell you as little as possible, close to useless information. If you are calling a third-party company, be aware that the person you get on the line has even less information on hand about you than your insurance company. In addition, the first person you speak to is a first level customer service person. The only information available to that person is your history of requests and authorizations as well as any status updates that have been entered into the database. Sometimes, the representative will have trouble finding you in the database if you don't have a case reference number for the request. In that case, your doctor's insurance authorization staff can help you retrieve a reference number.

Keeping these limitations in mind, just ask the initial question about reasons for denial. The person may or may not have any notes to his/her disposition. If you cannot get detailed information about the reasons for a denial, you have to ask for a supervisor. You should also ask questions about how the company operates. By operate I mean, what options are available to you and your physician before going into an appeal process. In general, I don't recommend appealing decisions before you have exhausted options like a physician-to-physician review (sometimes called peer-to-peer review) and resubmitting a request with additional information. The appeal process is cumbersome and takes a long time. It is much quicker to resubmit a request with additional clinical information than to appeal a coverage decision.

Ask questions like:

Is there a physician-to-physician review process?

What is the direct number that my physician can call to talk to the physician who makes the coverage decision? If any, which touch tone option should my doctor choose?

What is the deadline for such a review to take place? There is probably rule that a review has to be completed within a certain time from a denial or request for more information.

Sometimes there is a deadline, sometimes not. Some companies tell you about the option of a physician review, some don't. You don't want to miss out on this option, so ask the questions.

Can a time be scheduled by my doctor's office to accommodate the doctor?

What information will the doctor or his/her assistant need to have handy when calling in for the review?

If you really feel that you need more detailed information about the status and reasons for denial of a request, convince the representative that you need to speak to a supervisor or a clinical person who has the correct information.

Tip No. 4: Make a Physician Review Easy for Your Doctor

If a review process is available, make sure you provide your physician's assistant with all the necessary information. Your doctor is a busy person, so make it as easy as possible for him or her to complete the review. Provide the request/case/reference numbers and provide your date of birth so he or she doesn't have to look it up. Sometimes, the reference numbers are wrong and a date of birth is needed to identify the patient.

Provide the phone number and, if applicable, the touch tone option to get to the reviewing physician. Also, tell the assistant if there is a completion deadline. Give him or her as much information as possible on why the insurance company is denying the test or procedure, or what information is missing, so that your doctor has the necessary additional information readily available.

Sometimes, no information is missing, but it takes a specialist (your doctor) to explain why a test or procedure is needed. Most likely, the reviewing physician who makes the decision to cover or not won't be board-certified in orthopedics, radiology, pain management or any other specialty that applies. A specialist in geriatrics or obstetrics may well be making a decision on an orthopedic request. Often, the peer-to-peer reviews can be scheduled so your physician doesn't have to wait on the phone. Personally, I have had great success with reviews. I usually had to dig out the information myself, and inform all parties about what they need to do, but then the pre-authorization was always issued.

Tip No. 5: Avoid the Appeal Process

The appeal process is very cumbersome and has a long waiting time. If you discover that additional information is needed and can no longer be submitted because a request has already gone into denial status, ask you doctor's office to submit a new, more detailed request, to get your test more quickly. Processing a new request is typically a lot faster than an appeal. If that isn't possible, follow the instructions in the denial letter that your insurance company sent you.

If you have to appeal a decision, most states have a Consumer Health Assistance (CHA). You can find if your state already has one at www.healthcare.gov. The CHA can be extremely helpful in making your appeal as successful as possible. Make note of the timeline given in the denial letter. If you are going to ask for help from CHA, don't wait until the last minute, because the CHA offices usually have a heavy caseload.

11.2.3 Imaging and Diagnostic Testing

All the tips and suggestions given in the previous subchapter apply to imaging authorizations as well as procedures. When it comes to certain imaging studies there are additional challenges. Because insurance plans operate in different ways, I cannot give you specific advice, but will make some general suggestions.

If your imaging study involves any type of injection, make sure the injection was either pre-authorized or that it is covered without need for pre-authorization. I have been through the good and bad with insurance companies regarding imaging. I learned a lot from an episode in 2006. My sports doctor at the time had ordered a hip MRI arthrogram for me. During the arthrogram portion a radiologist injects contrast dye into your hip joint to help visualize the soft tissues inside the joint.

The imaging center called me to tell me that my MRI had been approved by my insurance company and scheduled me for the study. When I arrived at the imaging center, I found out that my insurance company had denied the injection portion of the study. I went ahead and let them perform the MRI, only to find out that the MRI was essentially useless to my doctor.

In a perfect world the imaging center should have informed me that the arthrogram had been denied, but their objective is to fill their timeslots and bill my insurance. I learned from this episode not only that I should be proactive about the entire authorization process, but also that I should always confirm with my insurance company that both the imaging study and the injection have been approved. In 2010, I had a different experience which another insurance company. I called to check if the authorization also included the injection. This time, the insurance company didn't care if I received an injection with dye or not; they simply didn't even consider an injection pre-authorization material.

11.2.4 Surgery

On January 1, 2011, three new CPT (Current Procedural Terminology) codes became effective and changed the road map regarding insurance coverage for surgery to treat FAI. Up to that point, each arthroscopy with osteoplasty and labral repair had to be billed as an unlisted procedure (CPT 29999) and getting the procedure approved and covered by insurance was more uncertain that it is now. The new CPT codes for osteoplasty and labral repair paved the way for many insurance companies to change their policies. Most insurance companies now cover surgery to treat FAI as well as labral repairs, but there are a few that still claim it is experimental.

The CPT codes in effect since January, 2011, used for arthroscopic osteoplasty and labral repair are:

29914: Hip arthroscopy, osteoplasty femur (CAM impingement)

29915: Hip arthroscopy, osteoplasty acetabulum (Pincer impingement)

29916: Hip arthroscopy, labral repair

Other surgical components, like iliopsoas release and labral graft, or open surgery have to be billed under different codes. The surgery protocol that your doctor's office submits to your insurance company after the procedure will describe the techniques and repairs used during surgery and the clinical findings in your joint. Even if you received a pre-authorization for a procedure, the last call on whether to reimburse your doctor is made after your insurance company has received the claim and surgery documentation from your medical provider. Keep in mind that insurance companies employ varying criteria that patients have to meet in order to establish medical necessity. For example, although five insurance companies say that they cover surgery to treat FAI and labral tears, what's required of your doctor to prove that you meet the criteria may be a little different for each insurance company. You can read up on the exact criteria in your insurance company's coverage position.

Even if you received a pre-authorization for a procedure, the last call on whether to reimburse your doctor is made after your insurance company has received the claim and surgery documentation from your medical provider.

Insurance plans work differently depending on if they are self-funded (the employer funds the insurance plan) or not self-funded. For self-funded plans, your company's benefits department regularly meets with the administrator of the self-funded plan. Those meetings can include decision making in individual coverage cases. No matter what type of insurance plan you have, your state's Consumer Health Assistance (CHA) can be very helpful in giving you the best opportunities to win an appeal or external review process. The CHA has channels and insurance contacts available to them that are not open to you as a member of the general public.

My first hip arthroscopy took place in January of 2011. In the process of obtaining authorization for the surgery, my doctor's office and I ran into problems, because the CPT codes that had just taken effect had not yet been adopted by my insurance company, and had not been uploaded into its database. In the process of sorting out the challenges, I learned that just because the American Medical Association has issued a CPT code and Medicare will start using that CPT code, individual insurance companies are not required to start covering procedures billed under those codes. Many companies are likely to follow suit with Medicare, but if an insurance company is not a Medicare provider in a particular state, the insurance company is not mandated to cover procedures under those codes or to automatically use the codes.

After numerous phone calls to my insurance company — during many of which I received false information — I finally found out that the new CPT codes were so new that they had not yet been uploaded into my insurance company's database. Therefore, the procedure couldn't be pre-authorized under the new codes. The doctor's office ended up resubmitting the request under the older unlisted procedure code. The coverage policy still read that labral repairs during hip arthroscopy were experimental.

I contacted the CHA in my state and received a great response. The CHA was able to contact a medical director for my insurance company directly and get the approval moving. Within a few hours, the medical director had called the reviewing authorization physician and my doctor's office to say that the procedures would be covered, despite the non-existence of the new codes in the database. From that point on, it was a breeze, at least insurance-wise. I have reason to believe that I was the first patient ever to get a labral repair covered by my insurance company, and I am just a little proud of that.

One thing that sometimes causes sticker shock and billing issues is anesthesia. The challenge occurs when it turns out that the anesthesiologist used during a surgery is out-of-network for your insurance plan. Most of us don't choose the anesthesiologist, so it is beyond our control to determine whether s/he is in-network or out-of-network. You can ask at your doctor's office whom your doctor likes to use for anesthesia, and check on that doctor's status with your insurance company.

If the damage is already done, you can often explain to the insurance company that the choice of anesthesiologist was out of your control, and the insurance company might reprocess the claim. If your insurance company still doesn't agree to process the anesthesiologist under your in-network benefits, the issue is worth a fight through your insurance company's appeals process, maybe with help of your state's Consumer Health Assistance.

In a worst-case scenario, if you cannot get your insurance company to cover the anesthesia, talk to the anesthesiologist's billing office and ask if they will treat the bill as if it were in network under your insurance plan. That is a bit tricky, because there is no contract with the insurance company and hence no contracted allowable rate. If you give your insurance company the name of an in-network anesthesiologist, they should be able to tell you how much the contracted rate would be for the billed procedure codes. Armed with that information, you might be able to settle on an amount owed that is much lower than the amount on the bill you received.

I am aware that the chapter on health insurance contains limited information to help hip impingement patients. Look for future books in the series of The Entrepreneurial Patient to find more detailed information on health insurance and administration.

12 MY STORY — CONTINUED

While finishing up this book, I am one year and two months out from the hip scope on my left hip. My hip joints are moving smoothly and I can walk a lot better and farther than I could before the surgeries. That is great improvement, considering I couldn't walk half a mile without severe pain, hip locking and catching. I still struggle with some muscle imbalances, but my gait is a lot better than it used to be. A lot of the buttock pain is gone. On some days, my iliopsoas gives me trouble. I can sit and write for hours at a time. I can shop and I can walk, but I struggle with exercise. Some of the groin pain has disappeared, but some remains. Now that I can distinguish the different pains from each other, I know that one kind of groin pain is gone and a different kind is still there.

As I have continued to work on *The Entrepreneurial Patient — A Patient's Guide to Hip Impingement,* I have also continued my medical quest to figure out why I still hurt. Two goals have been accomplished. This book is nearing its completion, and I have received a new diagnosis I can believe in — small, occult hernias in the groin. The pain came on in 2005, when I injured myself working out. Until recently, no orthopedic doctor — or other doctor for that matter — has managed to explain what is causing the remaining groin pain. In the process of interviewing surgeons to repair my hernias, I have heard different opinions.

Some surgeons don't believe there is a hernia if there isn't a bulge in the groin, and some believe hernias can be small and cause pain.

One of the opinions is that the difference between a sports hernia and a regular hernia is not significant and that the treatment for the two is the same. The opposite of that opinion is that a sports hernia is abdominal muscle weakness or tearing with a surgical treatment different than an inguinal or femoral hernia repair. I have been offered various treatment suggestions. Some surgeons don't believe there is a hernia if there isn't a bulge in the groin, and some believe hernias can be small and cause pain.

Since I have learned a lot along the way to both the hernia and the hip impingement diagnoses, I don't make decisions about surgery lightly. I will continue to do what an entrepreneurial patient should do. I will research and get multiple opinions from different doctors. When I feel comfortable, I will decide what method and which doctor will be the right choice for me. Right now I only feel comfortable with the diagnosis made by a hernia specialist based on an MRI, which shows small inguinal and femoral hernias only to the trained eye. Once I have settled for a surgeon and had the surgeries, I will start over with a different physical therapist to address remaining muscle imbalances and rebuild my core.

I hereby declare the arthroscopic surgeries to treat FAI a win, the physical therapy to rehabilitate after surgery to treat FAI a win, physical therapy to correct muscle imbalances caused by FAI only a semi-win, the hernia diagnosis a win and surgeries to treat the hernias an unknown. After seven years of health struggles, I am on the right track and very grateful for love, good decisions, patience, persistence and perseverance.

GLOSSARY

Acetabular fossa	Indentation located at the center (floor) of the hip socket.
Acetabular protrusion	The femoral head line crosses, or overlaps, the ilioischial line medially (toward the middle of the body) because the hip socket is too deep.
Acetabular retroversion	The front of the hip socket (acetabulum) is more lateral (to the side) than the back of the hip socket.
Acetabulum	The hip socket
Anterior	Front (example: front of pelvis)
Arthrogram	Injection of dye — contrast material — into a joint space to visualize the soft tissues of the joint on an MRI.
Articular cartilage	Joint cartilage
Bursitis	Inflammation of one or more bursae (small sacs) of synovial fluid.
CAM	CAM is an impingement lesion caused by excess bone, a bump, on the head/neck of the thighbone. It is sometimes described as a decreased offset of the femoral head-neck junction.
Cartilage	Cartilage is the tough but flexible tissue that covers the bone ends of a joint.
Cartilage debridement	Shaving off inflamed and frayed joint cartilage
Chondral defect	Injury or defect in the joint (articular) cartilage.
Chondrolabral junction	The contact area between joint cartilage and labrum
Coxa profunda	The acetabular fossa (indentation in the hip socket floor) overlaps the ilioischial line medially (toward the middle of the body) because the hip socket is too deep.
Coxa saltans	Snapping hip (iliopsoas impingement)

CT	Computed Tomography — allows for 3D-reconstruction of a joint.
Femoral anteversion	The neck of the thighbone leans forward in relation to the rest of the thighbone.
Femoral head	The ball-shaped head of the thighbone
Femoral head neck junction	The intersection of the ball and the narrower part of the thighbone called the neck.
Femoroacetabular Impingement	Hip impingement, FAI
Femur	The thighbone
Heterotopic ossification	Bone formation outside of normal bone structures.
Hip arthroplasty	Hip replacement
Hip joint capsule	The capsule around the hip joint consists partially of ligaments that surround and protect the joint.
Hypermobility	Lax ligaments that allow for a range of motion past the ordinary and/or predisposes a person to joint problems like FAI.
Labral debridement	A tear of the labrum is shaved away instead of repaired by means of sutures.
Labral repair	A tear of the labrum is repaired by means of sutures, also called anchors.
Labrum	A ring of soft, elastic tissue that follows the outside rim of the hip socket. Its suction effect holds the femoral head (ball) in place.
Lateral	Side (example: side of hip)
Ligament	A band of tough, fibrous and dense connective tissue that connects bones to other bones forming a joint.
MRI	Magnetic Resonance Imaging
Osseous structures	Wording used to describe bones in medical literature and radiology reports.
Osteoarthritis	A degenerative joint disease that causes joint inflammation and gradual loss of joint cartilage and wear on the underlying bone. Bone spurs and cysts may develop in the joint. FAI is thought to possibly cause osteoarthritis in the hip joints.

Osteoplasty	Bone shaving to remove CAM and pincer lesions.
Pathology	Disease or abnormality as it is seen on imaging, concluded by tests, labs and biopsies etc.
Pincer	Pincer in an impingement lesion caused by bone overhang or over-coverage from the hip socket.
Posterior	Back (example: back of thigh)
ROM	Range of Motion
Synovial fluid	Lubricating fluid produced when the joint is working, like biking.
Synovium	Joint lining
Tendinitis	Inflammation of tendons (soft tissue structures that attach muscle to bone)
Tendon	Soft tissue structures that attach muscle to bone
Tenotomy	Release or lengthening of a chronically tight muscle tendon. Common procedures for the iliopsoas and adductor longus tendons.

BIBLIOGRAPHY

1. **Hesch Institute.** What is the Hesch Method. *www.heschinstitute.com.* [Online] 2011. [Cited: February 6, 2012.] http://www.heschinstitute.com/our-method.html.

2. **Struan H. Coleman, MD, PhD.** Hip Mobility and Hip Arthroscopy: A Patient's Guide to Correcting Femoro-acetabular Impingement. *Hospital for Special Surgery.* [Online] 12 9, 2009. [Cited: 2 27, 2012.] http://www.hss.edu/conditions_Hip-Mobility-Arthroscopy-Patient%27s-Guide-Femoro-Acetabular-Impingement.asp.

3. *Clinical presentation of femoroacetabular impingement.* **Philippon, Marc J., et al., et al.** 2007, Knee Surgery Sports Traumatolog. Arthroscopy, Vol. 15, pp. 1041-1047.

4. **Banerjee, Purnajyoti and Mclean, Christopher.** Femoroacetabular impingement: a review of diagnosis and management. *Current Review Musculoskeletal Medicine.* 4, March 2011, 1, pp. 23-32.

5. **Taunton, Michael.** *Femoroacetabular impingment.* May 30, 2007. Orthopaedia Articles. In: Orthopaedia - Collaborative Orthopaedic Knowledgebase.

6. **Hanson, Chad.** *A Review of Femoroacetabular Impingement.* [interv.] Anna-Lena Thomas. Henderson, February 10, 2012.

7. **Muscolino, Joseph E.** *The Muscular System Manual. The Skeletal Muscles of the Human Body.* 3rd. Maryland Heights : Mosby Elsevier, 2010. pp. 1-8.

8. **Jerry Hesch, PT, MS.** [interv.] Anna-Lena Thomas. Henderson, March 15, 2012.

9. **Neumann, Donald A.** *Kinesiology of the Musculoskeletal System.* 1st. St. Louis : Mosby, Inc., 2002.

10. **Levangie, Pamela K. and Norkin, Cynthia C.** *Joint Function and Structure.* 4. s.l. : F.A. Davis Co., 2005. pp. 374-378.

11. *The Prevalence of cam-type femoroacetabular deformity in asymptomatic adults.* **Jung, K.A, et al., et al.** 2011, The Journal of Bone & Joint Surgery British, Vols. 93-B, pp. 1303-7.

12. *Do normal radiographs exclude asphericity of the femoral head-neck junction?* **Dudda, M, et al., et al.** 467, 2009, pp. 651-659.

13. *Clinical Presentation of Patients with Tears of the Acetabular Labrum.* **Burnett, Stephen R., et al., et al.** July 2006, The Journal of Bone and Joint Surgery, Vol. 88, pp. 1448-1457. 7.

14. **Douglas M. Gillard, DC.** Abnormal MRI in Pain Free People. *Chirogeek.com.* [Online] 2005. [Cited: March 2, 2012.] http://www.chirogeek.com/000_MRI-Abnormalities_Asymptomatic-Pats.htm.

15. *Hip Impingement: Identifying and Treating a Common Cause of Hip Pain.* **Kuhlman, Geoffrey S. and Domb, Benjamin G.** 12, December 15, 2009, American Family Physician, Vol. 80, pp. 1429-1434.

16. *Radiographic Predictors of Hip Pain in Femoroacetabular Impingement.* **Ranawat, Anil S., et al., et al.** 2011, Hospital for Specialty Surgery Journal, Vol. 7. 2.

17. *The diagnostic accuracy of acetabular labral tears using magnetic resonance imaging and magnetic resonance arthrography: a meta-analysis.* **Smith, Toby O., et al., et al.** s.l. : The European Society of Radiology, European Radiology, Vol. 21, pp. 863-874. 4.

18. *The role of arthroscopic thermal capsulorrhaphy in the hip.* **Philippon, Marc J.** 4, October 2001, Clinical Sports Medicine, Vol. 20, pp. 817-829.

19. *Groin Pain after Open FAI Surgery: The Role of Intraarticular Adhesions.* **Beck, Martin.** 3, March 2009, Clinical Orthopecic Related Research, Vol. 467, pp. 769–774.

20. *Acetabular Labral Tears: resection vs. Repair.* **Philippon, Marc J and Schenker, Mara L.**

21. *Treatment of Femoroacetabular Impingement: preliminary results of labral refixation.* **Espinosa, N, et al., et al.** May 2006, The Journal of Bone and Joint Surgery Am., Vol. 88, pp. 925-35.

22. *Arthroscopic debridement versus refixation of the acetabular labrum associated with femoroacetabular impingement.* **Larson, CM and Giveans, MR.** 4, April 2009, Arthroscopy, Vol. 25, pp. 369-76.

23. **Philippon, Marc.** *Clinical Research - Can Microfracture Produce Repair Tissue in Acetabular Chondral Defects?* 2008.

24. **Kelly, Bryan T.** Study Identifies Patients who Should not Undergo Surgery for Snapping Psoas Tendon. *Orthosupersite.com.* [Online] August 15, 2011. [Cited: March 15, 2012.] http://www.orthosupersite.com/view.aspx?rid=86618.

25. **John Hopkins Medicine.** Johns Hopkins Pediatric Orthopaedics. [Online] [Cited: March 16, 2012.] http://www.hopkinsortho.org/femoral_anteversion.html.

26. *Endoscopic management of the snapping iliopsoas tendon.* **Byrd, Thomas JW.** San Diego : s.n., 2009. Presented at the 28th Annual Meeting of the Arthroscopy Association of North America.

27. *Arthroscopic labral reconstruction in the hip using iliotibial band autograft: technique and early outcomes.* **Philippon, M J, et al., et al.** 6, June 2010, Arthroscopy, Vol. 26, pp. 750-756.

28. *IOC consensus paper on the use of platelet-rich plasma in sports medicine.* **Engebretsen, Lars, et al., et al.** 2010, British Journal of Sports Medicine, Vol. 44, pp. 1072-1081.

29. **Lundgren, Peter. Director, AKNA Institute, Sweden.** Dry Needling Course. *http://dryneedlingcourse.com.* [Online] 2010. [Cited: January 10, 2012.] http://dryneedlingcourse.com/what-is-dry-needling.

30. *Rehabilitation Exercise Progression for the Gluteus Medius Muscle With Consideration for Iliopsoas Tendinitis.* **Philippon, Marc J., et al., et al.** May 12, 2011, American Journal of Sports Medicine, Vol. 39, pp. 1777-1785. Published online before print on May 12, 2011.

31. **Philippon, Marc.** Optimizing Hip Rehabilitation with Computer Simulation. [Online] [Cited: April 30, 2012.] http://www.sprivail.org/optimizing-hip-rehabilitation-with-computer-simulation.

32. *Muscle recruitment patterns during the prone leg extension.* **Lehman, Gregory, et al., et al.** 3, 2004, BMC Musculoskeletal Disorders, Vol. 5.

33. **Dalton, Erik.** *Myoskeletal Alignment Techniques.* p. 36.

34. **Evidence Based Fitness Academy.** Synergistic Dominance of Hamstrings & Low Back Pain. *Evidence Based Fitness Academy's Blog.* [Online] January 23, 2011. [Cited: June 18, 2012.] http://blog.evidencebasedfitnessacademy.com/2011/01/23/synergistic-dominance--low-back-pain.aspx.

35. **Lehman, Greg.** The danger of hip extension - self care for labral tears. *www.thebodymechanic.ca.* [Online] 2012. [Cited: June 19, 2012.] http://thebodymechanic.ca/2010/01/28/the-danger-of-hip-extension/.

36. **Braun, Karina.** *Creating Peace with Your Hands.* 2nd. 2008. ISBN: 978-0-9816199-1-0.

37. **Zake, Yamuna.** Are you body logical? [Online] 2010. [Cited: April 25, 2012.] http://yamunabodyrolling.com/about/body_logic/.

38. **Roskopf, Greg.** The Science Behind MAT. [Online] [Cited: April 27, 2012.] http://www.muscleactivation.com/science.html.

39. *Femoroacetabular Impingment in the Athlete: Compensatory Injury Patterns.* **Voos, E. James, Mauro, S. Craig and Kelly, T. Bryan.** 2010, Operative Techniques in Orhtopaedics, Vol. 20, pp. 231-236.

40. *Experience with "sports hernia" spanning two decades.* **Meyers, William C, et al., et al.** 4, October 2008, Annals of Surgery, Vol. 248, pp. 656-665.

41. *Athletic Pubalgia and the "Sports Hernia": MR Imaging Findings.* **Zoga, Adam C., et al., et al.** 3, June 2008, Radiology, Vol. 247.

42. **Brown, William.** Understanding the Often Misunderstood and Misdiagnosed Sports Hernia. [Online] 2008. [Cited: April 17, 2012.] http://www.sportshernia.com/.

43. *Hip Disorders Up the Kinetic Chain: The Overhead Athlete.* **Kelly, Bryan T.** 2011. Current Concepts in Sports Medicine. Dr. Kelly works at Hospital for Special Surgery in New York.

44. *Hip Injuries in the Overhead Athlete.* **Klingenstein, G G., et al., et al.** March 14, 2012, Clinical Orthopaedics and Related Research.

45. *Acetabular labral tears following pregnancy.* **Baker JF, McGuire CM, Mulhall KJ.** 3, June 2010, Vol. 76, pp. 325-328. Sports Surgery Clinic and Mater Misericordiae University Hospital, Dublin, Ireland.

46. **American Medical Association.** About CPT®. *American Medical Association.* [Online] 2012. [Cited: January 11, 2012.] http://www.ama-assn.org/ama/pub/physician-resources/solutions-managing-your-practice/coding-billing-insurance/cpt/about-cpt.page?.

47. **U.S Department of Health & Human Services.** Consumer Assistance Program. *www.HealthCare.gov.* [Online] May 5, 2011. [Cited: January 11, 2012.] http://www.healthcare.gov/law/features/rights/consumer-assistance-program/index.html.

48. **Center for Medicare & Medicaid Services.** HCPCS Coding Questions. *Centers for Medicare Medicaid Services.* [Online] October 18, 2011. [Cited: January 11, 2012.] https://www.cms.gov/MedHCPCSGenInfo/20_HCPCS_Coding_Questions.asp.

49. **Active Release Techniques.** What is Active Release Techniques (ART) to Individuals, Athletes, and Patients? [Online] 2010. [Cited: April 26, 2012.] http://www.activerelease.com/what_patients.asp.

50. **Gurd, Vreni.** Walking, sacroiliac joint dysfunction and hip pain. *Trusted.MD.* [Online] Augtust 4, 2007. [Cited: March 2, 2012.] http://trusted.md/blog/vreni_gurd/2007/08/04/walking_and_sacroiliac_joint_dysfunction_and_hip_socket_degradation#axzz1nuzRQx6P.

FIGURES

Printed in Great Britain
by Amazon.co.uk, Ltd.,
Marston Gate.